Ethics, Conflict and Medical Treatment for Children

D1612568

Ethics, Conflict and Medical Treatment for Children

From Disagreement to Dissensus

DOMINIC WILKINSON, MBBS, BMedSci, MBioeth, DPhil, FRACP, FRCPCH
Professor of Medical Ethics, Director of Medical Ethics, Oxford Uehiro Centre for Practical Ethics; Consultant Neonatologist, John Radcliffe Hospital; Senior Research Fellow, Jesus College, Oxford, UK

JULIAN SAVULESCU, MBBS, BMedSci, MA, PhD
Uehiro Chair in Practical Ethics and Director, Oxford Uehiro Centre for Practical Ethics, University of Oxford, UK; Visiting Professorial Fellow in Biomedical Ethics, Murdoch Children's Research Institute; Distinguished Visiting International Professorship in Law, University of Melbourne, Australia

Forewords by
PETER SINGER
Ira W. DeCamp Professor of Bioethics, University Center for Human Values, Princeton University, USA; Laureate Professor, School of Historical and Philosophical Studies, University of Melbourne, Australia

NEENA MODI
Professor of Neonatal Medicine, Imperial College London; President, Royal College of Paediatrics and Child Health 2015-2018

ELSEVIER

Edinburgh   London   New York   Oxford   Philadelphia   St Louis   Sydney   2019

ELSEVIER

Notices

Practitioners and researchers must always rely on their own experience and knowledge in evaluating and using any information, methods, compounds or experiments described herein. Because of rapid advances in the medical sciences, in particular, independent verification of diagnoses and drug dosages should be made. To the fullest extent of the law, no responsibility is assumed by Elsevier, authors, editors or contributors for any injury and/or damage to persons or property as a matter of products liability, negligence or otherwise, or from any use or operation of any methods, products, instructions, or ideas contained in the material herein.

ISBN: 978-0-7020-7781-4

Content Strategist: Laurence Hunter
Content Development Specialist: Helen Leng
Content Coordinator: Deanna Sorenson
Project Manager: Julie Taylor
Designer: Ryan Cook

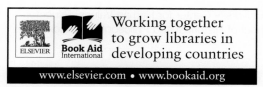

Working together
to grow libraries in
developing countries

www.elsevier.com • www.bookaid.org

your source for books,
journals and multimedia
in the health sciences

www.elsevierhealth.com

The
publisher's
policy is to use
**paper manufactured
from sustainable forests**

Printed in Poland
Last digit is the print number: 9 8 7 6 5 4 3 2 1

CONTENTS

In the field of bioethics, I am well known – some would say notorious – as a critic of the view that we should never intentionally take an innocent human life. Those who have heard about my views in bioethics often say that I am in favour of killing disabled babies. That's not accurate. I hold that the parents of infants born with severe disabilities should consult with their doctors about the prospects for their child. Then, if the parents decide that it is in the best interests of their child and their family for the infant to die, and the doctors consider this a reasonable decision, the doctors should be able lawfully to end the life of the child. At present, this is possible only in the Netherlands, and in very limited circumstances, in accordance with what is known as the Groningen Protocol.

Why then, in the case of Charlie Gard – an infant with a rare genetic condition that invariably leads to death before a child's first birthday – did I not support the doctors of Great Ormond Street Hospital? They went to court to prevent Charlie's parents from taking him out of the London hospital and flying him to the US for experimental treatment. The treatment, they told the court, had very little chance of saving Charlie's life. Allowing him to be taken abroad would, the doctors thought, only prolong his suffering. Pope Francis was on the side of the parents – and so was I, in a blog post I wrote with one of the co-authors of this book.[1]

No doubt some readers of that blog post were surprised to find that I was on the same side of this issue as the pope. But the assumption that I would side with the doctors rather than with the parents overlooked an important factor that, in my discussions of euthanasia for severely disabled infants, I have always insisted upon. It is for the parents to make the life or death decision for their child, unless their decision is manifestly contrary to the best interests of the child. The parents are the ones who will have to care for the child, if he or she survives.

This is a view I have held for many years. Helga Kuhse and I defended it in our 1985 book *Should the Baby Live?* Over the intervening years, parents of severely disabled infants have reinforced my thinking on this question. Among the more memorable is a letter I received shortly after I arrived at Princeton University in 1999. My appointment was on the front page of the *New York Times,* thanks to protests by prolife groups and a disability advocacy organization. The father of a severely handicapped child heard about the opposition to my views on euthanasia for severely disabled infants, and wrote:

> *'As the father of a severely handicapped son, I agree with you. He suffers from seizures every day, but the Catholic hospital that used extraordinary measures to keep his 24 week gestation, one pound, body alive without parental input does not care about him today. They got to play with their toys six years ago, and leave my family with the burden and David with the daily pain.'*

I support parents who judge it best that their child should die and want that death to be swift and humane; but for the same reason, I support parents who want their child to live, and want treatment that will give the child the best possible chance of survival. Not that the wishes of the parents override all other considerations. When it is clear that further treatment will cause the child pointless suffering because there is zero, or near-zero, chance of the child surviving anyway, the wishes of the parents for that further treatment should not prevail. Similarly, no one has a right to unlimited resources from the public healthcare budget. Resources are always limited, and

---

[1] Julian Savulescu and Peter Singer, 'Unpicking what we mean by best interests in light of Charlie Gard.' https://tinyurl.com/y9tzb9pe

intensive care beds used for one patient cannot be used for others. If it is obvious that the resources used to treat a child with very poor prospects could do much more good for other patients, then those resources should be used where they will do the most good.

Charlie Gard's situation was special in two important respects. First, it was not clear that Charlie would suffer if flown to the US. Perhaps his brain was so severely damaged that he was no longer capable of suffering. In that case, flying him to the US would not have done him any good as it could not have reversed the damage already done, but it would not have done him any harm either. If, on the other hand, he was still capable of suffering, then he could have been kept sedated during the journey and any subsequent treatment. So even if there were only a very small chance that the treatment would give Charlie a life worth living, from his own perspective, it would have been in his interests to take that chance.

Second, Charlie's parents were not asking for funding from the National Health Service for their son's travel and treatment. They received donations from well-wishers and supporters that were ample enough to pay for the travel and treatment. Thus, if the trip had done Charlie no good, it would not have wasted the resources of the National Health Service either. Moreover, it would have done one good thing: it would have allowed the parents the comfort of knowing that everything possible had been tried for their son. I cannot see a sufficient justification for the court to deny them that comfort.

Does this brief explanation of my views on the case of Charlie Gard leave you dissatisfied? If so, you have good reason for that. I have glossed over many important issues that cannot be explained in a few short paragraphs. What makes this book such an excellent analysis of life-and-death decisions in medicine is that it explores a range of perspectives on many of these challenging issues. That allows us to see why reasonable people differ over such decisions.

Where there is disagreement about important ethical issues, there is a temptation to seek consensus. We may try to persuade others to change their minds. For example, I have worked for decades to convince others that they should stop eating meat and donate more to help those in need in the developing world. We should acknowledge, however, that no matter how hard we try, we will not always succeed in persuading others that we are right. You may not agree with me about the Gard case, just as you may not agree with me about other ethical questions. Wilkinson and Savulescu, in their thought-provoking and thorough analysis of disputes about treatment for children, argue that we should embrace, not consensus, but dissensus. They suggest that, in the 21st century, the diversity of parental backgrounds, the complexity of medical science and the wide range of new and emerging treatments make disagreement more likely, and more likely to be intractable. They then propose a novel ethical framework for reaching decisions and acting on them, notwithstanding reasonable disagreements.

This book has something for general readers wishing to understand the background to cases that make tabloid headlines and will help to educate students of bioethics, but it will be especially challenging to those working at the cutting edge of medicine. It should stimulate discussions in paediatric and neonatal intensive care units everywhere. For a deeper understanding, read on.

Peter Singer
Ira W. DeCamp Professor of Bioethics,
University Center for Human Values,
Princeton University, USA;
Laureate Professor, School of Historical and Philosophical Studies,
University of Melbourne, Australia

Dominic Wilkinson and Julian Savulescu have written a thoughtful account about one family's personal tragedy, the story of Charlie Gard, a baby who became a cause celebre in 2017. Charlie's story was not new. Every day in many neonatal units around the world, doctors have to explain to parents and families that their child will not survive, or that if he or she does survive, it will be with profound impairment. Then – at least in the UK – a discussion takes place so that in the overwhelming majority of cases, parents and healthcare team come to a shared decision about what is best for the child and the family.

Stopping life support is not against the law in the UK if in the best interests of the child. The UK also pioneered palliative care, a great compassionate medical and nursing innovation. This recognises that withholding or withdrawing life-sustaining treatment does not mean withholding or withdrawing care. Good medicine encompasses the humane goal of helping a patient have a good death, and is about much, much, more than merely prolonging life.

The reaction of Charlie Gard's parents was also not new. They refused to accept that there was no possibility of cure. They refused to give up hope. Who could blame them? Initial denial of a painful reality is a human instinct, but with help, the majority of parents ultimately do accept. Around the world, the hearts of countless people went out to Charlie's parents because it seemed as though a cold legal process was tearing their child away from them. Many of these people should have known better. They should have realised that they were harming Charlie's parents by giving them false hope, and that they were harming Charlie, because the focus of his parents was not to help him to a good death, but instead was a futile quest to fight a reality they refused to accept. These people should have realised they neither knew the detail of the case, nor had the expertise to understand the medical implications.

I am a clinician and a researcher. I have had a fair amount of engagement with ethicists and appreciate they can help clinicians think through moral and ethical dilemmas with intellectual discipline. However, the buck does not stop with them, nor are they necessarily sufficiently familiar with what the brutal processes of living and dying can actually entail, or with the limitations of modern medicine. These are the responsibilities of clinicians. However, clinicians are human beings with differing perspectives, beliefs and biases. Of note therefore is that one of the main themes of the book is the idea of 'reasonable disagreement'. Conformity and uniformity are not what has driven human progress; rather, advance comes from a willingness to accept that divergent views are part of the human condition. I suggest it is neither rational nor desirable to expect agreement on issues of medical ethics.

This excellent and engaging book will help clinicians and ethicists, no less the lay public, appreciate there are no absolute truths in ethics. Ultimately, only constant reassessment, re-evaluation, and reflection will drive continued evolution of humanity's understanding of what is right.

Neena Modi
Professor of Neonatal Medicine, Imperial College London, UK;
President, Royal College of Paediatrics and Child Health 2015–2018

'They sought it with thimbles, they sought it with care;
They pursued it with forks and hope;
They threatened its life with a railway-share;
They charmed it with smiles and soap.'
The Hunting of the Snark, Lewis Carroll

Medical ethics is rife with argument.

At one level that can be a good thing.

Arguments and disagreements can be helpful in identifying ethical questions that need attention. After all, if everyone agrees about something, there isn't much to discuss. If people disagree, but do not care enough about it to argue, that probably means that it is a question that isn't very important.

Arguments are also a fundamental part of the methodology of ethics. When we are considering questions about what we ought to do, what should be done, arguments are important. We identify the reasons in favour of and against a particular course of action and try to critically appraise those reasons and weigh them up against each other. We can formally analyse the logic of a particular argument (is it valid, does the conclusion follow from the premises?), as well as scrutinise the premises (are they true?).

However, sometimes all this argument in ethics can seem like a problem. That can be because of an impression that philosophers or ethicists will argue about anything. (How many philosophers does it take to change a lightbulb? That depends on how you define 'change'. Or 'lightbulb'. Or 'philosophers'.) Other times, ethical debates can seem intractable, bound to end in stalemate. For any ethical question of substance, it can seem like there are arguments on both sides (and proponents of each), with no way of ever reaching a resolution. Some people find all this argument upsetting and wish that it were possible to identify solutions without confrontation.

As philosophers with a medical background, we have often participated in academic ethical debate. We have also, though, seen the way that these debates play out in the wards and in the lives of families. We have participated in meetings with other health professionals where there has been disagreement (sometimes heated) about what would be best for a seriously ill patient. We have had long discussions with families and patients who had different views from us about medical treatment that they wanted or did not want. We have also sometimes been on the other side of the desk and found ourselves arguing with doctors about treatment for ourselves[2] or for a family member.

We have collaborated professionally for more than a decade and have common views on many ethical issues. In early 2017, though, as a dispute about medical treatment for a seriously ill child started to receive attention in the media, we found ourselves on opposite sides of the debate. We wrote a series of blogs advancing the case in support of and against continued intensive care and experimental treatment. We wrote a pair of contrasting editorials for the leading English medical journal *The Lancet*. As the legal case advanced through a series of appeals, we continued to argue

[2]Savulescu, J., (2003). Festschrift edition of the Journal of Medical Ethics in honour of Raanan Gillon. *J Med Ethics,* 29, 265-266; Savulescu, J. (2018). Wicked Problems, Complex Solutions, and the Cost of Trust. *J Med Ethics,* 44(3), 147-148.

and to disagree about what the right course of action would be. With time, the key areas of disagreement and agreement between us became clearer.

The process of argumentation can often be helpful in understanding what is at stake in an ethical debate. Sometimes when two people have different opinions on a topic, it can be useful to listen to a discussion between them. That can give the listener an appreciation of the competing points of view and help them to identify their own perspective. In ancient philosophy, this process of reasoned dialogue between opposing speakers was referred to as a *dialectic*. (Plato's famous written account of Socrates' conversations with various other Athenians is a prime example.) The dialectical approach was seen by the ancients to be a key way of making progress in philosophy. As we discussed and debated the Gard case, we found a greater understanding of the opposing point of view, and were led to reflect on, reconsider and sometimes temper our own views.

However, our thinking about the case also led us to wider issues. We reflected on the ethical implications of disagreement: what should we do as society in the face of diverging viewpoints about treatment for a child? In the 21st century, this problem seems to be an urgent one for medical ethics. There are ever-expanding options for treatment, from those that are mainstream, through those that are in development, to some that are untested and merely offer a hypothetical benefit. The complexity and scale of the information that is now available – both to health professionals and to families – means that reaching a common understanding about the trajectory of illness and its treatment is increasingly challenging. Moreover, our societies are becoming, in many parts of the world, more diverse, with families and patient from very different ethnic, cultural and religious backgrounds all seeking treatment within a common health system. The search for consensus and agreement seems doomed.

Yet, perhaps we can agree to disagree? It seemed to us that if we could understand the boundaries of reasonable disagreement, we could find a way to resolve disputes without requiring all to agree on vexed value-laden decisions.

This book is the result. It starts with a paradigm example of disagreement, the tragic case of Charlie Gard. The court case arose because of apparently irresolvable disagreement between a family and health professionals about what would be best for a child. In the first chapter, we outline the details of the case, summarising some of the key arguments that played out in the courtroom and the events that followed.

In the second part of the book, we explore in more detail the central ethical issues that led to disagreement in the Gard case and in other cases of disputed medical treatment. Our aim is to move beyond the specific features of Charlie's case to clarify and shed light on the questions relevant to other children and future cases. We will seek, where possible, areas of common ground. We will focus especially on children in this book, though most of these issues are relevant to patients of any age. Disputes about children's treatment seem to arise and reach the courts more commonly than for adults. These disputes are also particularly difficult to resolve (for example, they often can't be settled by asking what the patient wants or would have wanted). We also concentrate especially on treatment in intensive care – as, again, these fraught life-and-death decisions are where disagreement seems to be most common, and one of us (DW) is a practising neonatal intensive care specialist in Oxford – but the general lessons can apply to other types of treatment, too.

In Chapter 2, we analyse what it means to say that a treatment is 'futile'. We identify several different ways that this term might be understood and argue that it is rarely able to provide a clear basis for health professionals declining to provide treatment. Paradoxically, increasing sophistication of medical technology and diagnostic information (for example, genomic information) can make it harder, rather than easier, to know when a treatment will not work.

We then move, in Chapter 3, to explore the question of whether treatment would be in a child's best interests. We look at the reasons or arguments that are sometimes thought to count against prolonging a child's life with medical treatment; for example, because a child is suffering, because her future life is reduced in quantity or quality or because she has a reduced chance of survival. Some of these provide stronger or clearer reasons not to prolong life, while others are subject to more reasonable disagreement.

In Chapter 4, we move away from the interests of the individual to the important question of limited healthcare resources – particularly in a public healthcare system. We will look at how this question is relevant to issues relating to provision of life-prolonging treatment in intensive care, and some of the challenges in deciding how or when to limit treatment on the basis of distributive justice concerns (e.g., when providing treatment to one patient would potentially cause harm to others). This again is becoming more challenging and more difficult with medical advances and new possibilities for treatment.

In Chapter 5, we look at a topic that seems very familiar in ethics – that of the ethical challenges that arise in research. We will focus, though, not on the usual issues about the design of trials, or the process of consent or the role of ethics committees. We will concentrate on issues such as what level of harm is sufficiently low that it is ethical to enrol a noncompetent child in a trial, and whether it is ethical (and if so, when) to test new or experimental treatments on gravely ill and dying children.

Finally, in the last chapter in this section of the book (Chapter 6), we look at the role of parents in decisions about treatment for children. Why isn't it, in the end, up to a child's parents whether he or she has continued life support or embarks on experimental treatment? That will include examining a very contemporary challenge: treatments available overseas that are not supported or provided locally. When should such medical tourism for children be permitted or prohibited?

In the third part of the book, we will try to draw some lessons from the Charlie Gard case and other treatment disputes for medical ethics in the 21st century. We describe a general approach (Chapter 7) to controversial medical treatment decisions that builds on dissensus rather than on consensus. We argue that reasonable disagreement is a sign of moral uncertainty, and that where this is present, decisions should usually be based on the values of the patient (or parents), rather than those of doctors.

In Chapter 8, we argue in favour of a two-level model for decisions that separates out questions of resources from questions of the interests of the child. We propose treatment review panels that could assess these different questions separately and suggest that this approach could allow decisions to be made in a way that is faster, less adversarial and more respectful of different viewpoints than the existing court-based model for resolving treatment disputes.

Finally, we will come full circle and return to the case that started our reflection. In Chapter 9, we will apply the model that we have developed to a similar (hypothetical) case of disagreement about intensive care and experimental treatment – in a child with severe spinal muscular atrophy. Our aim is to show how agreement could be possible, despite diverging perspectives and points of view. We also include, at the end of the book, a pair of appendices that set out what we each feel are the strongest arguments for and against treatment for Charlie Gard. We continue to disagree about what should have happened in that case. However, as we argue through the book, disagreement is not always a bad thing.

This book is being published by Elsevier as a companion publication to our forthcoming textbook *Medical Ethics and Law: a curriculum for the 21st century*.[3] That book (co-authored with Jon Herring) sets out core ethical and legal topics for health professionals in training and in practice. Readers of this book who are interested to learn more about some of the issues in this book (for example, ethical issues and decisions at the end of life, research ethics and regulation,

---

[3]It will be a complete revision of the highly successful standard medical textbook: Hope, T., Savulescu, J. and Hendrick, J. *Medical ethics and law: the core curriculum.*

resource allocation) can find more material there, as well as an overview of some other cutting edge ethical issues for our times, including genethics, neuroethics and information ethics.

Before we move to the substance of the book, we should note some important points about aims and limitations. This is a book of ethics rather than a book of law. We aim to analyse the ethical issues, rather than the specific legal questions. We have drawn heavily on the official reports from several cases that ended up in the courts; however, our reason for doing so is that such reports provide rich and detailed information about the reasons and arguments in cases of disagreement. We have made some recommendations for how disagreements should or could be arbitrated. There is a further question (beyond the scope of our expertise and of this book) about whether our suggestions are compatible with existing law, and whether or how the law should be changed. We have concentrated, for the most part, on cases from the UK. This is partly because of our familiarity with those cases, but also because of the ready availability of court judgments relating to cases in this jurisdiction. However, the general points that we make about disagreement and about processes for dealing with it are relevant internationally.

The reliance on court judgments (and media reports) also points to a significant limitation of our analysis. We have relied entirely on publicly accessible information about the Charlie Gard case and the other cases that we discuss. We did not have any input from either the families or the health professionals involved in these cases. In such cases, while the judgments are helpful, they are not a complete record of all the ethically salient features of cases. There may be other facts about the cases that would change our mind about them. Our conclusions about specific cases must be conditional. That also highlights one prominent feature of the Gard case that we will not explore in depth in this book. The Gard case occurred in an era of social media and global media that saw enormous public scrutiny of the family and health professionals. It also encouraged editorialists, politicians and the public to reach conclusions about the case, often with only partial information about the medical and ethical issues at stake. There are serious questions about how to manage and navigate mainstream media, social media and political agendas when private ethical dilemmas reach the public space. However, we will have to leave those issues for others to address.

Finally, it is vital to pay tribute to the children, families and health professionals who find themselves or have found themselves at the centre of disputes about medical treatment. It is all very well to discuss ethical theory, but disputes in medicine are about real illnesses, real suffering and real people. There are few things in life that are more stressful than having a child with a life-threatening illness. Families or health professionals are, in almost all cases, trying desperately to make the best decision that they can in extremely difficult circumstances. When they find themselves in conflict, the impact on all parties can be overwhelming. For the reasons that we have summarised above, and elaborated through this book, such disagreements are inevitable. The only thing that we can change is how we deal with them. We will argue that, while current approaches have some strengths, there is a better, fairer way.

DW
JS

ACKNOWLEDGEMENTS

This book was only possible because of the support of several organisations and individuals.

We would like to first acknowledge the support of the Uehiro Foundation on Ethics and Education and their President, Mr Tetsuji Uehiro. Without their support, there would be no Chair of Practical Ethics at the University of Oxford, nor Centre for Practical Ethics. We are deeply grateful for their support since 2002, which has made this book possible through the creation of positions at the University of Oxford, as well as its ongoing support of the Centre.

We would like to thank the editors of *The Lancet* for their circumspect and timely treatment of our contributions to the Charlie Gard case.

JS is grateful to the Murdoch Children's Research Institute for providing him with a Visiting Professorial Fellowship in Biomedical Ethics. Much of the work relating to this book was done during his 4-month period spent there between July and October, 2017. He benefitted greatly from discussions with a range of experts in related areas, and is especially grateful to Bob Williamson, David Thorburn and John Christodolou. JS also benefitted from a concurrent Visiting Professorship at the University of Melbourne and is grateful to Judge Julie Dodds-Streeton for very helpful discussions.

JS and DW have benefited greatly from the support of the Wellcome Trust through research awards that have contributed to this research [WT106587/Z/14/Z, WT 104848/Z/14/Z]. More recently, the Wellcome Centre for Ethics and the Humanities has provided a platform for presentation of work and ideas, as well as valuable research support [WT203132/Z/16/Z].

DW would like to thank Jesus College, Oxford, for a senior research fellowship and for allowing him the privilege of writing in the beautiful secluded environment of the Fellows' library. He would also like to thank the nursing and medical staff at the newborn care unit of the John Radcliffe Hospital for their patience and forbearance while he was working on this manuscript and for their brilliant teamwork in caring for critically ill newborn infants and their families.

We would especially like to thank Rocci Wilkinson and Miriam Wood for tireless personal, administrative and research support, and for running the blog (blog.practicalethics.ox.ac.uk) which supported so much of our contemporaneous discussion.

DW
JS

Disagreement

CHAPTER 1

The Charlie Gard case

'Begin at the beginning and go on till you come to the end; then stop.'
Alice in Wonderland, Lewis Carroll

Shortly after three o'clock on the 28th of July 2017, in a private room of a specialised hospice in suburban London, staff disconnected the breathing machine that was keeping alive 11-month-old infant Charlie Gard. Lying on either side of him, his parents Connie Yates and Chris Gard held his hands, leaned close and talked to him. They spoke to him of how proud they were of him. They saw him open his eyes briefly, and close them. Minutes later Charlie's heart stopped, and he was gone.[1]

This was the conclusion – quiet, private and fleeting – to a dispute about medical treatment that had been none of those things. In the preceding 4 months, a protracted series of court hearings around disputed treatment for Charlie Gard had yielded global media attention and an outpouring of sympathy from onlookers around the world. It had attracted statements of support from many public figures, including US President Trump and the Pope.

Charlie's parents had been seeking experimental treatment that might improve his rare genetic condition. They had raised funds for him to travel to the US, where a medical specialist had offered to provide treatment. Many observers could not understand why the doctors at London's Great Ormond Street Hospital opposed the requested treatment. Many found it hard to see why the UK and European courts[a] had decided against Charlie's parents and authorised withdrawal of life support.

In the final stages of the court hearing, 3 days before he died, Chris and Connie accepted the view of experts that medical treatment could no longer help him, and that it was time to allow him to die. Their own medical experts from overseas had examined Charlie and concluded that his condition was now too far advanced for experimental treatment to work. The family agreed to a plan to withdraw life support, though bitterly regretted what they perceived as a lost chance to help Charlie.

But how had it reached this point? Where did the disagreement come from, and why had this decision been a matter for the court in the first place?

In this first chapter, we will describe the background to the Charlie Gard case and how it played out over the first half of 2017. We will look at how decisions about medical treatment are normally made, and the role of the court in decisions. We will outline some of the important ethical questions raised by the Gard case that will form the basis for the rest of this book.

The Charlie Gard story

Charlie Gard was born, apparently healthy, in West London in August 2016. His parents, Chris and Connie, enjoyed a normal first few weeks with him at home. However, at a few weeks of

---

[a]We will refer in this book to 'UK courts', but it is worth acknowledging that there are some differences between courts in different parts of the UK. Most cases of disputed medical treatment relating to children have been referred to the courts of England and Wales.

age, his parents started to notice that he wasn't able to lift his head as well as other children, an early sign of muscle weakness. By a couple of months of age, he was losing weight and muscle strength, and Charlie was admitted to the specialist children's hospital at Great Ormond Street, where soon afterwards he was put on a breathing machine in intensive care because he was not strong enough to breathe for himself. Doctors suspected that he had a genetic condition affecting his muscles and brain. A biopsy of his muscle and, later on, whole genome sequencing, identified the cause as an extremely rare condition with a long technical medical name: 'infantile onset encephalomyopathic mitochondrial DNA depletion syndrome' (MDDS for short).

There are a number of genetic disorders that can cause worsening muscle weakness in babies. Some of these are problems with the structure of muscles. Others are problems with nerves, nerve signals or the brain.

MDDS is a condition that affects the basic energy structures of the body, the mitochondria. Mitochondria are found in most cells in the human body. There are several hundred in each human cell, and perhaps as many as 10 quadrillion in the whole human body. The energy released by these mitochondria fuels much of the activity of cells. They are often compared to batteries, but mitochondria are much more complicated than batteries. One little-known feature is that they contain their own genetic material or DNA. One theory is that they were originally bacteria captured by our primitive ancestor cells. Mitochondrial DNA is separate from the main chromosomes that we inherit from our parents (which live in the nucleus of the cell). It is much smaller than nuclear DNA. Nevertheless, these mitochondrial genes have essential roles in energy production and in regulating other important cellular processes.

Normally, mitochondria are continuously making more mitochondrial DNA. They do this by synthesising and by recycling the basic building blocks of DNA (nucleosides) and then assembling them in a way that copies the existing mitochondrial genes ('replication'). This continuous process of replicating mitochondrial DNA is essential for the mitochondria to work properly. In some very rare genetic conditions, however, there are mistakes (mutations) in the instructions that tell the cells how to make the mitochondrial DNA building blocks or how to put them together. This leads to the cells having much lower amounts of mitochondrial DNA than normal – this is the problem that affected Charlie Gard.

There are different forms of MDDS, but all typically cause progressively worsening energy production problems in the body. As an analogy, it is a little bit like a problem with your mobile phone battery. Your phone might start out working fine; however, over time, the charge seems to run out very quickly, and the battery does not last long before running out of power. In the case of a mobile phone, you might be able to get a new battery – but of course it isn't possible to replace billions of mitochondria.

The specific genetic form of MDDS that Charlie Gard had (affecting a gene called *RRM2B*) had previously only ever been reported in 15 cases in the world. All of these babies had early onset of muscle weakness and rapid progression of symptoms, and died within a few months.[2] This form of MDDS is called 'encephalomyopathic'. The muscles do not work properly because of a lack of energy, while the effect on the brain leads to a lack of brain growth and seizures.

By the time that doctors had diagnosed Charlie's condition, he was paralysed and unable to breathe without a machine. He was found to have congenital deafness, and his heart, liver and kidneys were affected by the disorder. As this diagnosis became clear, doctors at Great Ormond Street felt that the outlook for Charlie was extremely poor and started to talk to his parents about whether continuing to keep him alive on life support was the right thing to do. In November, there was a meeting of the clinical ethics committee at Great Ormond Street to discuss whether Charlie should have surgery to perform a tracheostomy. This is a procedure that creates a hole in the front of the neck so that a breathing tube can be passed directly into the windpipe (trachea), rather than being inserted through the nose or mouth. This surgery is performed for patients who are receiving long-term invasive breathing support from a machine. At that meeting, the ethics committee heard evidence from doctors. They felt that Charlie's quality of life was so poor that 'he should not be subject to long term ventilation'[b] The ethics committee supported the medical team's assessment that Charlie should not have a tracheostomy.

There is no cure for MDDS and no proven treatment for Charlie's severe form of the illness. However, Charlie's parents, understandably, found this news very difficult to accept. His mother took to the internet to research possible treatments that might be in development or used in other parts of the world. In that research, she found mention of a treatment that had seemed to help some children with a less severe form of MDDS. She was in contact with a parent in the US whose child had received that treatment, and Connie Yates asked the specialists at Great Ormond Street if they would try it for Charlie.

The problem for Charlie's mitochondria was a lack of the building blocks that he needed to make new DNA inside his mitochondria. But what if he were given a supplement containing those building blocks? Could that bypass the problem and help his cells to make more mitochondrial DNA?

That is the basic idea behind the treatment that Connie Yates found on her search of the internet. 'Nucleoside therapy' (also called 'nucleoside bypass therapy') has been used in children with a different genetic form of MDDS. *TK2* is another gene that causes depletion of the mitochondrial DNA. The *TK2*-related form of MDDS is also rare, but it has been described in more than 50 children.[2] In this condition, the problem is not in making new DNA building blocks (nucleosides) – it is in the genes that recycle old nucleosides. Because cells are continuously making mitochondrial DNA, they need to be very efficient at recycling and reusing the building blocks from old strands of DNA. There are two basic types of nucleosides, called purines and pyrimidines. In the *TK2*-related form of MDDS, there is a problem with recycling the pyrimidine nucleosides. This causes less severe problems than the *RRM2B*-related form – children develop weak muscles in their first 1 or 2 years of life (rather than in the first weeks or months, as in Charlie's illness). They too can have problems with muscle strength, affecting their ability to move, feed and breathe. However, it does not usually affect the brain as much. Children with the *TK2*-related form of MDDS have, in the past, usually died in early childhood, though some have survived longer, even into adulthood.[2]

Arturito Estopinan is one of those older survivors. In 2012, when Arturito was age 1, doctors in the US diagnosed him with the *TK2*-related form of MDDS. His parents were told that there was no medical treatment, and that he would likely die within months.[3] However, just like Charlie Gard's parents, the Estopinans combed the internet and contacted experts across the US looking for something that might help him. They spoke with one expert, Professor Michio Hirano, a neurologist in New York who had been experimenting with a new treatment in mice that had a disease similar to the *TK2*-related form of MDDS. Arturito was the first person to receive nucleoside treatment, and a year later he was able to come home, while still receiving intensive medical care and breathing support. In July 2017, Arturito's father described some of the improvements in muscle strength they had seen with the nucleoside therapy: 'They have allowed him to get stronger by moving his arms, his fingers, his legs. He's even trying to move his hips'.[4] Arturito remained severely disabled, and dependent on a ventilator to breathe. But he was alive, and, rather than worsening, he had improved to some degree. This improvement has also been seen in research studies. In mice genetically engineered to have a form of *TK2*-related MDDS, early supplementation with the pyrimidine nucleosides apparently led to higher mitochondrial DNA levels and less severe clinical features.[5] It wasn't a cure, but it seemed to help.

---

[b]Para 59. Details here and below are taken from the High court judgment, with paragraph numbers cited for specific quotations. The full judgment is available at http://www.bailii.org/ew/cases/EWHC/Fam/2017/972. html Great Ormond Street Hospital v Yates & Ors [2017] EWHC 972 (Fam) (11 April 2017).

Connie Yates had found Arturito's story when she was researching Charlie's condition. She contacted Arturito's parents, who put her in contact with Dr Hirano. If nucleoside therapy could help in *TK2*-related forms of MDDS, could it work in Charlie's form, involving *RRM2B*? Dr Hirano could not give a definite answer. Nucleoside treatment had not been tested, either in animals or in humans with the *RRM2B*-related form. The genetic defect in this condition is more severe, and giving the same pyrimidine nucleosides that help in the *TK2*-related form would not be enough. In theory though, giving a combination of three different nucleosides might work. Dr Hirano told Connie that it could be worth a try given how serious Charlie's condition was. At the request of Charlie's parents, Dr Hirano corresponded at the end of December with the mitochondrial specialist at Great Ormond Street. The specialist asked Dr Hirano a series of questions, which were later reported in one of the court judgments:

> Question 1: 'What is the evidence that this treatment might help?'
> Dr. Hirano's response: 'There is no direct evidence, but there is a theoretical scientific basis for saying it could.'
> Question 2: 'Could the drugs cause toxicity?'
> Dr. Hirano's response: 'The only toxicity seen is dose-related diarrhoea'.
> Question 3: 'As the drugs do not cross the blood-brain barrier, is there any possibility of efficacy in a child with an epileptic encephalopathy?'
> Dr. Hirano's response: 'This had been previously suggested in published research, but there is theoretical and anecdotal evidence that the drugs could in fact cross this barrier and, therefore, have effect on the brain. In particular, TK2 patients who have been treated have not developed seizures or encephalopathies as had those who were not treated.'
> Question 4: 'If we were to embark on a clinical trial, how long would you suggest, and what outcome measures?'
> Dr. Hirano's response: 'A 3-month trial should be sufficient.' [He suggested a range of non-invasive outcome measures.][c]

The third question was important to the doctors at Great Ormond Street because there were worrying signs that Charlie's brain was affected by MDDS. In the middle of December, Charlie had started to have epileptic seizures. Since he was paralysed, there were not always outward signs of these seizures. However, electrical tracings of his brain (an electroencephalogram, EEG) had shown a combination of frequent seizures, as well as abnormal background electrical activity. These findings together indicated a brain that was very sick (epileptic encephalopathy). Moreover, the Great Ormond Street doctors were concerned that nucleoside therapy would not reach the brain because of the protective blood-brain barrier.

Dr Hirano was supportive of trying nucleoside therapy. Given that, the Great Ormond Street specialist started to arrange for Charlie to receive the treatment. This was an untested and unlicensed medicine, and to be able to provide it would require special approval. The decision was referred back to the ethics committee at Great Ormond Street, with a meeting planned for the 13th of January. There was a provision for Charlie to have a tracheostomy on the 16th of January.

However, the meeting and the surgery did not go ahead. In early January, the doctors arranged further tests of Charlie's brain. This included a magnetic resonance imaging (MRI) brain scan on the 6th of January. This was essentially normal and showed only subtle changes, a finding that is apparently typical in MDDS because the basic problem is at the microscopic level (and so is not visible on scans). A repeat EEG, though, on the 10th of January, was felt to again show signs that Charlie's brain was severely affected by MDDS, with frequent electrical seizures and a pattern of severe epileptic encephalopathy.

---

[c]Para 76, High Court judgment.

On the 13th of January, doctors at Great Ormond Street met with Charlie's parents and told them that the trial of nucleoside therapy would not go ahead. All of the medical teams at the hospital involved in Charlie's care had agreed that this treatment would be 'futile, and would only prolong Charlie's suffering'.[d]

There had been some disagreement between Charlie's parents and the doctors at Great Ormond Street since November, but by this meeting in January, it seemed clear that the medical team and Charlie's parents had very different views about what would be best for him. Charlie's parents were determined that life support should continue and that Charlie should receive a trial of nucleoside therapy. His doctors, though, felt that it was wrong to continue to keep Charlie alive. They felt that he was suffering by being kept alive by machines in intensive care, and that nucleoside treatment had no hope of helping him.

How often do disagreements like this occur in intensive care units? How are they usually resolved?

Approximately 2000 children die in paediatric and neonatal intensive care units each year across the UK.[e] Some of these children die suddenly, with little warning. In many cases though, a child is seriously ill and, sadly, death is expected. In paediatric and neonatal units, somewhere between two-thirds and three-quarters of deaths follow decisions to either stop life support or not to attempt resuscitation if a child deteriorates (we will refer to these together as 'end-of-life decisions').[8–10] There are different reasons why treatment might not be provided, but, fundamentally, the concern is that continuing treatment or trying to resuscitate would not help, and would do more harm than good. That might be because, even with treatment, the child would survive for only a short time (quantity of life). Or it might be because the child could survive, but would do so with a very reduced quality of life. We will return to discuss those reasons in more detail in Chapters 2 and 3.

Across the country, then, as many as three or four times every day, there are decisions made about life support for children or babies. Those decisions, in the vast majority of cases, are made jointly by families and health professionals. Parents or carers, together with the doctors and nurses looking after the child, come to a shared view that certain types of potentially life-prolonging treatment are not right for the child. That is not to say that these decisions are easy, or are made lightly. Quite the opposite: these are often agonising decisions, made only after much soul-searching, and after all other options have been considered and rejected. The point is rather that conflict and disagreement are not an inevitable or even a usual part of end-of-life decision-making for children. In almost all cases, while decisions are difficult and distressing, they are able to be reached with the agreement of all those caring for the child – both professionals and family.

But how often is there disagreement? It is hard to know. One study in the Netherlands interviewed health professionals caring for 147 newborn infants who had died after an end-of-life decision. In about one in ten cases (18 infants), the doctors reported that there had been conflict between the professionals and parents.[11] Many of those cases were ones where the infant was predicted to be severely disabled if they survived (these are quality of life reasons – see Chapter 3). However, in all of the 18 cases, agreement was eventually able to be reached. Sometimes this occurred after the parents obtained a second opinion. Sometimes it was after the child's condition worsened and parents changed their mind. In some cases, a compromise was reached where treatment would not be withdrawn but resuscitation would not be provided if or when the child's heart stopped. A 2016 Canadian study of 942 babies who died asked doctors about end-of-life decisions that had been made. From almost 800 cases where there had been discussions about end-of-life treatment, doctors reported that it had been 'difficult' to reach agreement in only 12% of cases.[12]

---

[d]Para 83.
[e]In England and Wales, there are approximately 650 deaths in paediatric intensive care units a year.[6] There are another 1400 newborn infants who die each year across the UK.[7] A high proportion of these deaths are likely to occur in neonatal units.

A study of neonatal units in London provides some additional insight. This study reported the outcome for 68 seriously ill infants where there were discussions about end-of-life decisions. In half of these cases (34 babies), parents and professionals reached a decision to stop treatment or not resuscitate after an initial meeting. In the other half, treatment continued and there were further discussions, often including second opinions. In 16 of these cases, there was eventually agreement to limit treatment, while in the other half, treatment continued.[8]

Protracted disagreement is the exception rather than the rule. There were no cases in any of those studies where doctors were reported to have obtained legal advice or gone to court. But where parents and health professionals cannot reach agreement, there is the option of going to the court to resolve the impasse. One report suggests that, in 2016, UK courts were asked to make decisions about medical treatment for a child in 18 cases.[13] However, not all of those cases will necessarily have been about end-of-life treatment. (For example, some may have been cases where parents disagreed between themselves about treatment, or where parents wished to refuse treatment – e.g., blood transfusions for religious reasons.) From published court records, it appears that there were five end-of-life treatment disagreement cases in the first half of 2017. They included:

1. An 11-year-old boy with advanced bone cancer that had spread to his lungs. Doctors wished to provide palliative care; parents did not agree with his diagnosis, and were opposed to him being provided with palliative care. (Court decided in favour of providing palliative care.)[14]

2. An 8-month-old girl with inoperable complex congenital heart disease. Doctors did not wish to provide resuscitation (including inserting breathing tubes and other invasive measures). Parents accepted that her life was limited, but wished her to receive resuscitation. (Court decided in favour of withholding resuscitation.)[15]

3. A 13-year-old child with severe multiple disabilities (severe cerebral palsy, scoliosis, intellectual disability, epilepsy, poor lung function). Doctors did not wish to provide invasive life-prolonging treatment (including resuscitation, mechanical ventilation and renal dialysis), and wished to provide palliative care; mother was opposed to any limitation of treatment. (Court decided in favour of providing palliative care.)[16]

4. An emergency court hearing about a 3-month-old infant who had deteriorated after surgery for a large subdural haematoma and was thought to have a very poor prognosis. Parents sought a court order to prevent doctors from limiting treatment; doctors wished to not provide further neurosurgery, resuscitation or escalation of treatment. (Court decided in favour of no further surgery or resuscitation.)[17]

The fifth case was Charlie Gard.

After the meeting in January, it was clear to Charlie's parents that Great Ormond Street would not provide him with nucleoside treatment. Connie and Chris started to look at other options, and on the 30th of January they started an online appeal to raise funds for him to travel to the US for treatment. They estimated that it would cost £1.2 million for Charlie to be treated in the US.

Meanwhile, Charlie's doctors obtained a series of second opinions from intensive care specialists, neurologists, lung specialists and mitochondrial specialists at other hospitals in the UK. They also obtained an opinion from a mitochondrial research team in Barcelona with specific expertise in MDDS.

On the 24th of February, lawyers for Great Ormond Street Hospital applied to the Family Division of the High Court seeking the court's permission to withdraw the artificial breathing support keeping Charlie alive, to provide him with palliative care and to not provide nucleoside treatment. There was a brief hearing in early March that was adjourned to allow Charlie's parents to gather evidence from overseas experts and present them to the court.

In the first week of April, the court heard evidence from Charlie's parents, from experts at Great Ormond Street and from the US expert Dr Hirano, who gave evidence by telephone. As is usual in such cases, there was a court-appointed guardian who was tasked with representing Charlie's interests in court. The following week, on the 11th of April, Justice Nicholas Francis gave his decision.

We will summarise here the basic elements from that judgment, since they set out issues that we will return to in later chapters.

Legal principles

The first part of Justice Francis' judgment set out the legal principles underpinning his decision. As noted in the preface, our focus in this book is on ethical questions rather than on legal questions. Nevertheless, an appreciation of the key legal principles will help understand the decisions that were made for Charlie Gard. They will also provide a starting point for some of the ethical questions that we will return to in later chapters.

1. The court in the UK has legal authority to make decisions in a child's best interests.

   The judge noted:

   'Some people might ask why the court becomes involved at all, why should the parents not be the ones to decide? A child's parents having parental responsibility have the power to give consent for their child to undergo treatment, but overriding control is vested in the court exercising its independent and objective judgment in the child's best interests.' (para 11)

   Obviously most of the time, and for most medical decisions, courts are not part of treatment decisions for children. The court is asked to make a decision either if there is no one to make a decision for a child (e.g., if the child is orphaned, or if parents are unable or unwilling to decide) or if there is disagreement about the decision. As indicated above, in rare instances health professionals and families cannot agree on what would be best for a seriously ill child. In that circumstance, the UK approach is neither to assume that the doctors know best, nor that parents are making the right decision. As in many other areas of life, when there is intractable disagreement between different parties about something important, there is a need for an impartial arbiter – the court is asked to decide. The court is then asked to determine what would be best for the child. This is sometimes referred to as the 'best interests' of the child.

2. What is best for a child does not always mean prolonging life.

   Courts in the UK, as in other parts of the world, have traditionally been very cautious about making decisions that would lead to the death of a patient. The judge quoted a decision in the case of Charlotte Wyatt (another young child whose parents and doctors disagreed about treatment)[18]:

   'There is a strong presumption in favour of a course of action which will prolong life, but that presumption is not irrebuttable.' (para 13)

   In other words, prolonging life is important, but it is not always the right thing to do. This vital interest could be outweighed 'if the pleasures and the quality of life are sufficiently small and the pain and suffering or other burdens of living are sufficiently great'. (para 39)

3. The best interests of a child include more than just medical factors.

   Medical evidence about illness and treatment is important, but court decisions in past cases have understood a child's (or older patient's) interests to incorporate a range of elements. For example:

   'These include … medical, emotional, sensory (pleasure, pain and suffering) and instinctive (the human instinct to survive) considerations.' (para 39)

4. The views and opinions of parents should be carefully considered.

   Parents are important because of their knowledge of the child:

   'Where, as in this case, the parents spend a great deal of time with their child, their views may have particular value because they know the patient and how he reacts so well.' (para 39)

They are also important because of the child's interest in their relationship with their parents. Their wishes 'may illuminate the quality and value to the child of the child/parent relationship'. (ibid)

However, courts in the UK have not considered parental wishes to be directly relevant to the child's best interests: 'Their own wishes, however understandable in human terms, are wholly irrelevant to consideration of the objective best interests of the child.' (ibid)

We will return shortly to the evidence heard by the court, but it is worth noting here that the first three principles are not particularly controversial, and are reflected (to a varying extent) in legal decisions about medical treatment for children in many different countries.

However, the last of the previous four points is more distinctive, in that it identifies a distinctly limited role for parents in assessing the best interests of a child. It is this factor that perhaps explains why the UK is relatively unique in its legal approach to disputed treatment for children. As noted in the quotation from the judgment, parental wishes do not carry much weight for the court in consideration of the best interests of the child. It has meant that, unlike elsewhere, the UK courts have been prepared to make decisions to authorise withdrawal of medical treatment against the objections of parents.[f]

In the US, by contrast, courts have been very reluctant to override parents who desire potentially life-prolonging medical treatment for their child.[19] This has proved true even in extreme cases such as that of Baby K (an infant with anencephaly who received mechanical ventilation for a prolonged period)[20] or that of the Californian girl Jahi McMath, in which a court had ruled the child was 'legally dead'.[21]

After summarising the legal basis for the decision, Justice Francis summarised evidence presented by the hospital and by Charlie's parents. That evidence related to two issues relevant to the decision for Charlie: his current quality of life and the benefit of nucleoside treatment. A third important issue, that of the cost of treatment, was considered not to be relevant.

A. Quality of life.

The court heard evidence from various medical experts about Charlie's current medical state. They indicated that he was dependent on a mechanical ventilator as he had no ability to breath on his own. He could no longer move his arms or legs, and had no spontaneous movement of his fingers, hands, toes or feet. He was no longer able to open his eyes enough to be able to see. Because of his genetic condition, he was deaf. The intensive care consultant at Great Ormond Street indicated that repeated EEG tests had shown that he was 'persistently encephalopathic' – he was not brain dead, but there was no sign of normal brain responsiveness.

One of the doctors who examined Charlie reported seeing no movement apart from a flicker of Charlie's lips in response to pressing on his fingers. A nurse from the intensive care unit, who had spent over 200 hours at Charlie's bedside over several months, reported that she had not seen him grasp fingers. Because of his lack of movement and response, she felt that it was impossible to tell if Charlie was awake or asleep.

Charlie's parents had a different view about Charlie's brain function. They felt that he knew when his parents were present and could experience pleasure (e.g., tickles). They reported that he sometimes tried to hold their hands and open his eyes. They could tell the difference between when he was awake and asleep.

There were different views about whether or how much Charlie was experiencing pain or discomfort from the treatment he was currently receiving. The bedside nurse who gave evidence reported that it was 'impossible to know' if Charlie suffered pain or experienced

---

[f]This might also explain the role of the court-appointed guardian in Family Court proceedings. In cases like Charlie Gard's, the court appoints a separate independent party for the child who has a specific role to safeguard the child's interests. For an older child, the guardian has an independent role in assessing the wishes of the child.

pleasure. His parents felt that there were things that he did not like (such as nasal suction or a blood test), which they could tell because his heart rate would go up. The medical team gave evidence that the treatments that Charlie required to stay alive (being on a ventilator, having his airway suctioned) could cause pain. The mitochondrial expert at Great Ormond Street testified that it could not be demonstrated that Charlie experienced pain, but that it was possible. The medical team apparently believed that he was suffering: 'She said that she did not regard his pain of being of a low level of suffering, but something more significant.' (para 114)

Despite their different perspectives, both the medical experts and parents appeared to agree that Charlie's current quality of life was poor. The medical team had apparently felt, even before Charlie developed seizures, that 'his quality of life was so poor that he should not be subject to long-term ventilation'. His parents indicated: 'We would not fight for the quality of life he has now... This is not the life we want for Charlie.' (para 110)

B. Nucleoside treatment

Given apparent agreement that Charlie's current state was not one that should be prolonged with life-sustaining treatment, the key issue was whether the proposed nucleoside treatment would or could change that.

The court heard evidence about nucleoside treatment in patients with the *TK2*-related form of MDDS. Dr Hirano reported that a group of international experts (including himself) had treated 18 patients with the *TK2* form of MDDS with nucleoside treatment. Patients had gained weight on treatment. All were still alive. Some had improved in strength.

The nucleoside treatment had never been tried in animals or in humans with the *RRM2B*-related form of MDDS, so its effect could not be predicted. There was a scientific rationale for the treatment, and (in the patients with the *TK2* form) it appeared to have few side effects. The only side effect was diarrhoea if given in too high a dose. It was also very cheap. Because it was relatively easy to administer and low risk, the central question was whether it would work (and whether this would justify continuing intensive care for a period of months more).

Could nucleoside treatment work in Charlie? One important difference between the two forms of MDDS is that the *RRM2B* form affects the brain, while the *TK2* form affects (mostly) the muscles. Dr Hirano indicated that nucleoside treatment could cross the blood-brain barrier, and potentially work in the brain. This was based on previous research experience in the *TK2*-related form of MDDS. The Great Ormond Street expert, in contrast, indicated that there was no evidence in humans that the nucleoside treatment could enter the brain.

The other central issue for Charlie was whether he already had sufficient brain damage that the nucleoside treatment could not help him. When he had first spoken with the medical team at Great Ormond Street, Dr Hirano had indicated that Charlie should have an MRI brain scan, as 'severe brain involvement' would mean that treatment should not be tried. As noted earlier, that MRI had not shown any major changes; however, the development of very abnormal electrical activity had led doctors at Great Ormond Street to believe that he had severe brain involvement by MDDS. After reviewing recent EEGs, Dr Hirano indicated to the court: 'I can understand the opinion that he is so severely affected by encephalopathy that any attempt at therapy would be futile. I agree that it is very unlikely that he will improve with that therapy.' However, he also felt that he could not rule out some benefit. The probability was low, but not zero. 'I think to a large extent it is irreversible, but I cannot say it is completely irreversible.' (para 118)

C. Costs of treatment

One issue that was raised briefly in the judgment, but dismissed, was the question of the cost of treatment. Charlie's parents had sought funding to allow Charlie to travel to obtain nucleoside treatment overseas, as it was clear to them that the public health system in the UK would not provide treatment. By the time of the court hearing in April, their fundraising campaign had reached its target of £1.2 million. However, the judge indicated that 'funding was never an issue'. Great Ormond Street had been prepared to provide nucleoside treatment to Charlie, but had changed their mind once he deteriorated and they felt it would not help him. The judge wrote:

'It is imperative that I make clear that this case is not about money and, if anyone were to suggest that Charlie would have nucleoside treatment but for the cost, they would be completely wrong.'

(We will later respectfully disagree, at least in part, with this statement; see Chapter 4.) One of the important roles of ethical analysis in complex cases is to separate out questions of fact from those of value. The factual questions are going to be based on evidence, and scientific and medical experts are important in determining those. However, questions of value are not going to be determined by evidence in the same way. To address those, we will need careful ethical and philosophical analysis.

What were the key questions of fact in the Charlie Gard case? Table 1.1 summarises the main ones and identifies areas of disagreement.

TABLE 1.1 ■ Factual questions and contrasting perspectives in the case of Charlie Gard

Factual questions	Hospital	Parents/Parental experts
What was Charlie's level of awareness/cognition?	Charlie was encephalopathic. He did not appear to respond or interact.	Charlie was aware of his parents' presence. He could respond to them and experience pleasure.
How much did he experience pain/suffer from intensive care?	It was not possible to be sure, but doctors believed that Charlie was suffering.	Charlie appeared to respond negatively to some medical procedures.
What was the chance of improvement in Charlie's encephalopathy or myopathy?	Charlie had irreversible brain damage. A 'tiny theoretical chance'. 'No chance'.	Parents: 'We truly believe that these medicines will work'. Expert: Main benefit would be improvement of weakness. Brain damage is to a large extent irreversible, but not definitely irreversible. Probability is low but not zero. 'Only a small chance of meaningful brain function'.
How long would treatment need to be provided to determine if he has any improvement?		3 months.
What is the best function that he could achieve with treatment?	Likely to continue to deteriorate, to remain immobile and to have severe cognitive impairment.	If his seizures were controlled, he could interact, smile, look at objects and use hands.
Could he be ventilator-independent with treatment?	No.	Possibly reduced time on ventilator.
How long could he live with continued life-sustaining treatment?	Not known/not discussed.	

We divide the opinions into the hospital and the family. The legal guardian appointed to represent Charlie's interests largely concurred with the medical opinion about facts and ethical questions and concluded that 'it is not in Charlie's best interests to travel to America to receive nucleoside therapy'. For simplicity, we will not discuss the guardian's perspective separately.

'It is with the heaviest of hearts but with complete conviction for Charlie's best interests that I … rule that Great Ormond Street Hospital may lawfully withdraw all treatment, save for palliative care, to permit Charlie to die with dignity.' (para 23)

Charlie's parents cried out in dismay and wept as the judge read out his decision in open court. The judge provided a detailed justification for his conclusion. He had been convinced by the medical experts at Great Ormond Street that nucleoside treatment would be futile. By this he meant 'pointless or of no effective benefit'. He noted that the US expert Dr Hirano had conceded that the treatment was very unlikely to benefit Charlie. Justice Francis observed that there was agreement from all parties, including Charlie's parents, that his current quality of life was so poor that it was not justified to prolong it without hope of improvement. He ruled that nucleoside treatment should not be provided, and that doctors could proceed with their plans to withdraw life-sustaining treatment from Charlie.

Legal appeals

After the April decision in the High Court, there were a series of legal appeals. Fig. 1.1 shows schematically the current available options for resolving a disagreement about treatment for a child in the UK.

In most cases, a single court might be involved. In the Gard case, all possible legal appeals were pursued. The decision was reviewed in the Court of Appeal (initial decision upheld, 23rd May), Supreme Court (declined permission to appeal, 8th June) and European Court of Human Rights (endorsed approach of UK courts, 20th June). All of those courts ultimately supported the initial decision that it would be in Charlie's best interests to stop life support and not provide nucleoside treatment.

We are not going to review those court judgments in detail here. Much of the evidence presented at those court hearings repeated what had been discussed at the High Court. (In the UK, appeals courts typically allow appeal on the basis of claims of errors of law or of the judicial process. They do not usually reassess the factual evidence presented and debated at the lower court. The Supreme Court will usually only allow appeals if there is a legal principle of general public importance at stake.) Much of the legal appeals therefore turned on points of law; for example, questions of the jurisdiction of the court, or whether the High Court decision contravened elements of the European Convention on Human Rights. We will set aside those questions for legal scholars to debate elsewhere.

However, there was some discussion of two questions that are of clear ethical relevance.

HARM THRESHOLD

One of the grounds for the first legal appeal focused on when courts may override parental wishes. We noted previously that the UK court becomes involved in decisions about medical treatment if parents and doctors cannot agree on what would be best for the child. However, Charlie's parents argued in the Court of Appeal that this is the wrong standard. Their lawyers claimed that 'the court may not interfere with a decision by parents in the exercise of their parental rights and responsibilities with regard to their child's medical treatment, save where *there is a risk the parents' proposed course of action may cause significant harm.*'[22] (para 54) [emphasis added]

One of the arguments of the legal team drew an analogy with the legal approach to placing children in care. The UK Children Act (2004) sets out when public authorities can remove a child from their parents. Social services in the UK can obtain a court order only if *'the court is satisfied that the child concerned is suffering or is likely to suffer significant harm, and that the harm, or likelihood of harm, is attributable to parental care or the child being beyond parental control.'*[23]

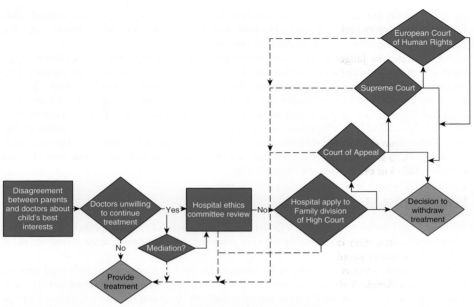

Fig. 1.1 Current approach to resolving disagreement about medical treatment for a child in the UK. This figure relates to situations where parents wish for continued treatment that doctors do not believe would be in child's interests. Solid arrows indicate path towards withdrawal of treatment in face of parental opposition. Dotted lines indicate a path towards provision of treatment. Resolution may be possible at earlier stages if parents and doctors reach agreement.

The idea is that public authorities cannot intervene for a child any time that they feel that parents are doing less than the best for their child. All of us who are parents know, if we are honest, that we are not perfect, and there will be some times and some decisions where we do less than the best possible for our children. Perhaps that is because we have several children, and doing the best for one child means doing less than the best for another. Perhaps it is because our own work or our own interests are important too, and sometimes they take priority. Perhaps it is just because we all have times when we are tired, stressed, overworked, distracted or just human, and fail to live up to the high standard of 'doing the best' for our children – much as we might aspire to that.

The invocation of 'significant harm' in the Children Act means that the state gives parents some leeway – it acknowledges that they have a right to care for their children in the way that they choose – within limits.

But if the 'harm threshold' is the standard for the state intervening in parental everyday decisions – shouldn't that also apply to medical decisions? Charlie's parents' legal team suggested that in cases where parents have an alternative viable treatment option to that proposed by doctors, the test should not be whether one of these is 'better'. Instead, the parents' wishes should be overridden only if their preferred treatment plan would be harmful.

That was the argument put to the Court of Appeal. The judges in that court ultimately rejected that legal argument. As a point of law in the UK, medical treatment cases are treated differently from decisions about when local authorities can take over the care of a child.

That still leaves the ethical question unanswered – *should* we use the harm threshold for deciding when parents' wishes about medical treatment should be respected or refused? If we think the answer to that is right, it may be that the law should change. We will argue in Chapter 8 that the harm threshold is the right way to set out the boundaries of parents' discretion about medical treatment.

As an aside, the judges in the Court of Appeal indicated that, even if Justice Francis had been required to use a significant harm test rather than a best interests test, he would likely have reached the same decision.

FREEDOM TO TRAVEL

One of the arguments discussed in the European court hearing was whether the previous court decisions not to allow Charlie's parents to take him overseas for treatment deprived him of his liberty. Article 5 of the European Convention on Human Rights grants everyone a right to liberty and security. It gives individuals a right not be arrested or detained without an appropriate legal basis. In the press, it was claimed that the court decisions had effectively 'imprisoned' Charlie in Great Ormond Street.[24]

The specific legal claim about imprisonment was rejected by the European Court. (In essence, the convention does not stop countries from detaining individuals – it stops countries from detaining people without good legal reason, process and safeguards. The court felt that the reasons, process and safeguards articulated and followed by the UK courts meant that Charlie's Article 5 rights were not being violated.) However, the wider ethical question is one that we will return to. Particularly for cutting edge treatments, it is not unusual for treatment to be available in some countries but not others. Travel for treatment (so-called 'medical tourism') is becoming increasingly common. When should, or shouldn't this be permitted?

The final appeal

After the European Court rejected his parents' appeal, it appeared that the final legal avenues for Charlie's parents had been exhausted. It seemed to all external observers that it was no longer a question of if treatment would be withdrawn from Charlie, but when.

However, the public and media attention to Charlie's case did not wane. In the last week of June and first week of July, there were countless headlines, opinion pieces and comments as global attention focused on Charlie's plight. There were several very high profile statements of support. On the 2nd of July, Pope Francis released a statement indicating that he hoped that 'their desire to accompany and care for their own child to the end is not ignored'.[25] A day later, US President Trump tweeted: 'If we can help little #CharlieGard, as per our friends in the U.K. and the Pope, we would be delighted to do so.' Later that week, a number of international medical and scientific experts came forward offering to provide treatment (in hospitals in New York or Rome) and offering apparently new evidence allegedly increasing the chance of benefit from nucleoside treatment. On the 10th of July, Great Ormond Street Hospital elected to bring this evidence back to the High Court.

Over a series of hearings from the 10th July until the 24th, Justice Francis again considered Charlie's case. The court heard further testimony from Dr Hirano by videoconference, and the judge then arranged for the US specialist to review Charlie in person in London, as well as for further tests. The next week, several specialists (including Dr Hirano, but also other international experts) took part in a multidisciplinary meeting. Following that meeting, further tests were arranged to assess the severity of Charlie's illness, including a full body MRI. On the 24th of July, Connie and Chris appeared in court and withdrew their appeal against the medical and legal decisions; they now accepted that further treatment could not help Charlie. Treatment was withdrawn later that week.

Cases like Charlie's offer an insight into the ethical dilemmas facing parents, doctors and courts. We have summarised in some detail the Charlie Gard case to provide the basis for further ethical discussion. We have explained some of the legal process and reasoning (though the law is not our main focus). We have also tried to put this extraordinary case into the broader context of most end-of-life decisions, as well as other cases of disagreement between parents and doctors.

Our aim in the next section of the book is to move beyond the specific details in Charlie's case. In doing so, our analysis will shed some light on disagreement itself – on its moral significance in culturally and ethnically diverse societies, and its implications for policy and practice. It is not surprising if difficult cases about providing or withholding life-prolonging treatment divide experts and communities.

References

1. Smith-Squire, A. (2017) Our last hours with our son. *Daily Mail*. Accessed from: http://www.dailymail.co.uk/news/article-4762390/Charlie-Gard-s-parents-hours-son.html.
2. El-Hattab, A. W. & Scaglia, F. (2013) Mitochondrial DNA depletion syndromes: review and updates of genetic basis, manifestations, and therapeutic options. *Neurotherapeutics*, 10, 186-98.
3. Gebelhoff, R. (2015) Family carves out its own path in fight against 4-year-old's rare disease. *Washington Post*. Accessed from <https://www.washingtonpost.com/national/health-science/family-carves-out-its-own-path-in-fight-against-4-year-olds-rare-disease/2015/09/04/7d18d8b0-2c91-11e5-a5ea-cf74396e59ec_story.html?utm_term=.53490173263c>.
4. Knight, V. (2017) His son tried the experimental treatment Charlie Gard's parents want. *CNN*. Accessed from <http://edition.cnn.com/2017/07/18/health/american-baby-treatment-charlie-gard-case/index.html>.
5. Lopez-Gomez, C., Levy, R. J., Sanchez-Quintero, M. J., Juanola-Falgarona, M., Barca, E., Garcia-Diaz, B., et al. (2017) Deoxycytidine and Deoxythymidine Treatment for Thymidine Kinase 2 Deficiency. *Ann Neurol*, 81, 641-652.
6. Plunkett, P. & Parslow, R. (2016) Is it taking longer to die in Paediatric Intensive Care in England and Wales. *Arch Dis Child*.
7. MBRRACE-UK. (2016). 'Understanding babies' deaths in the UK: 2014.' From <https://www.npeu.ox.ac.uk/downloads/files/mbrrace-uk/reports/MBRRACE-UK-PMS-Report-2014-Infographic-poster.pdf>.
8. Aladangady, N., Shaw, C., Gallagher, K., Stokoe, E. & Marlow, N.; for Collaborators Group (2017) Short-term outcome of treatment limitation discussions for newborn infants, a multicentre prospective observational cohort study. *Arch Dis Child Fetal Neonatal Ed*, 102, F104-F109.
9. Hellmann, J., Knighton, R., Lee, S. K., Shah, P. S. & Canadian Neonatal Network End of Life Study, G. (2016) Neonatal deaths: prospective exploration of the causes and process of end-of-life decisions. *Arch Dis Child Fetal Neonatal Ed*, 101, F102-F107.
10. James, J., Munson, D., DeMauro, S. B., Langer, J. C., Dworetz, A. R., Natarajan, G., et al. (2017) Outcomes of Preterm Infants following Discussions about Withdrawal or Withholding of Life Support. *J Pediatr*, 190, 118-123.e4.
11. Verhagen, A. A. E., de Vos, M., Dorscheidt, J. H. H. M., Engels, B., Hubben, J. H. & Sauer, P. J. (2009) Conflicts about end-of-life decisions in NICUs in the Netherlands. *Pediatrics*, 124, e112-9.
12. Hellmann, J., Knighton, R., Lee, S. K., Shah, P. S. & Canadian Neonatal Network End of Life Study, G. (2016) Neonatal deaths: prospective exploration of the causes and process of end-of-life decisions. *Arch Dis Child Fetal Neonatal Ed*, 101, F102-F107.
13. Doward, J. & Robertson, H. (2017) Ten cases like Charlie Gard's heard in English courts this year. *The Observer*. Accessed from <https://www.theguardian.com/uk-news/2017/jul/29/ten-cases-like-charlie-gards-heard-english-courts-this-year>.
14. *An NHS Trust v SK (Best Interests Decision -Palliative Care)* [2016] EWHC 2860 (Fam) (04 November 2016).
15. *Great Ormond Street Hospital for Children Foundation NHS Trust v NO & KK & Ors* [2017] EWHC 241 (Fam) (14 February 2017).
16. *A Local Authority & Anor v MC & Ors (Care proceedings)(Inherent Jurisdiction)* [2017] EWHC 370 (Fam) (24 February 2017).

17. *An NHS Hospital Trust v GM & Ors* [2017] EWHC 1710 (Fam) (30 June 2017).
18. *Portsmouth NHS Trust v Wyatt* [2005] 1 F.L.R. 21.
19. Paris, J. J., Ahluwalia, J., Cummings, B. M., Moreland, M. P. & Wilkinson, D. J. (2017) The Charlie
    Gard case: British and American approaches to court resolution of disputes over medical decisions. *J
    Perinatol*, 37, 1268-1271.
20. New York Times News Service (1994) Court says doctors must treat Baby K, infant born without
    most of brain. *Chicago Tribune*. Accessed from <http://articles.chicagotribune.com/1994-02-20/news
    /9402200448_1_periodic-respiratory-crises-anencephalic-babies-active-labor-act>.
21. Luce, J. M. (2015) The uncommon case of Jahi McMath. *Chest*, 147, 1144-1151.
22. *Yates & Anor v Great Ormond Street Hospital For Children NHS Foundation Trust & Anor (Rev 1)* [2017]
    EWCA Civ 410.
23. *The Children Act*, 1989. https://www.legislation.gov.uk/ukpga/1989/41/section/31.
24. Mendick, R. (2017) Charlie Gard is being held 'captive' by the NHS, complains the family's spokes-
    man. *The Telegraph*. Accessed from <http://www.telegraph.co.uk/news/2017/07/12/charlie-gard-held
    -captive-nhs-complains-familys-spokesman/>.
25. *Vatican Radio*. (2017, July 3, 2017). 'Pope Francis expresses closeness to Charlie Gard's parents.' From <http://
    en.radiovaticana.va/news/2017/07/03/pope_francis_expresses_closeness_to_charlie_gard's_parents/1322731>.

PART II

Agreement

CHAPTER 2

Futility

'They went to sea in a Sieve, they did,
In a Sieve they went to sea:
In spite of all their friends could say,
On a winter's morn, on a stormy day,
In a Sieve they went to sea!'
The Jumblies, Edward Lear

'Accordingly, the entire highly experienced UK team, all those who provided second opinions and the consultant instructed by the parents in these proceedings share a common view that further treatment would be <u>futile</u>. For the avoidance of any doubt, the word "<u>futile</u>" in this context means pointless or of no effective benefit'. (para 93)
'the prospect of the nucleoside treatment having any benefit is as close to zero as makes no difference. In other words, as I have already said, it is <u>futile</u>.' (para 119)
JUSTICE FRANCIS 11 APRIL [EMPHASIS ADDED]

'there is a distinction between the medical definition of <u>futility</u> and the concept of <u>futility</u> in law .... Medicine looks for "a real prospect of curing or at least palliating the life-threatening disease or illness from which the patient is suffering", whereas, for the law, this sets the goal too high in cases where treatment "may bring some benefit to the patient even though it has no effect on the underlying disease or disability".... In the present case, tragically, this is a difference without a distinction in the light of the judge's finding that the potential benefit of nucleoside therapy would be "zero".' (para 44)
JUSTICE MACFARLANE COURT OF APPEAL 23 MAY [EMPHASIS ADDED]

'Futile' is a word that comes up a lot when there are disagreements over treatment between patients (or their families) and doctors.

One way of understanding these disagreements is as a clash between two fundamental principles in medical ethics. The first of these (beneficence) says that doctors must act to help or heal patients. The second principle (autonomy) says that doctors must respect patients' desires (at least those that reflect their most important values). But these principles can sometimes suggest opposite actions. What should the doctor do when what the patient wants would not do any good, or would be harmful? In the past, doctors made decisions about what was in the best interests of their patients. This is called paternalism. Hard or strong paternalism is when doctors make decisions on behalf of a competent person who could decide for herself. Soft or weak paternalism is when they make those decisions when the patient has some flaw or problem in her own decision-making process, e.g., she is confused or delirious.

In a more paternalistic era, doctors would simply not discuss or offer treatments that they felt would not benefit the patient. They believed that they knew best; patients by and large did not protest, or they did not know enough to protest. In more recent decades, there has been a shift in the doctor-patient relationship to emphasise the ethical importance of the values of the patient. There has also been an enormous increase in the number of available treatments, some of which (but not all of which) are beneficial. In combination, these changes have enormously increased the potential for conflict.

Moreover, there is growing acknowledgement of 'value pluralism': that there may a range of reasonable sets of values. Some people may prioritise living longer, others having a better quality of life. Some people value high risk/high pay-off options, others security. Increasingly, doctors are confronted with patients with a range of different values, and in some cases, those are not conventional.

The specific term 'futility' first appeared in medical ethics in the 1980s. The idea was that if doctors identified that a particular treatment was 'futile', this would solve the problem of conflicts. Doctors had no obligation to provide futile treatment, and so it wouldn't be paternalistic if they refused to do so. Or so the argument went.

In the next decade, many physicians and ethicists sought to define 'futile treatment' in a way that would be practically applicable. For example, US physician Lawrence Schneiderman proposed that treatment could be labelled futile if it had not worked in the last 100 cases, or if the patient would be permanently unconscious or dependent on intensive medical care.[1] Yet there were also critics. Robert Truog and colleagues, writing in the *New England Journal of Medicine* in 1992, argued that 'the concept of futility obscures many ambiguities and assumptions'.[2] Brody and Halevy, 3 years later, suggested that the attempt to define futile treatment was itself futile; the available definitions did not succeed in justifying unilateral withholding of treatment.[3] By 2000, some ethicists observed what they perceived to be a concept in terminal decline.[4]

As the quotations from the Charlie Gard case make clear, however, futility has not gone away. It continues to be part of legal and ethical discussion around disputed medical treatment. In this chapter, we will look at two reasons why, in cases like that of Charlie, the concept of futile treatment is unhelpful. We look first at the problem of definition – it is very difficult to reach agreement on a clear (and applicable) definition of the term. We will then look at a bigger problem. Even if it is possible to reach agreement on a definition, it is rarely possible to determine with confidence when that definition applies. Paradoxically, this problem is actually made more difficult by advances in medical information and medical technology.

Language

Before trying to define futile treatment, it is perhaps worth noting some related concepts. Because 'futility' has been so heavily criticised, there has been a tendency for recent guidelines to avoid the word and use other terminology instead. There are a range of synonyms that have been suggested (Box 2.1).

Some of these terms may be preferable to the word futility, because of their connotations. For example, a number of these indicate that they are medical determinations – identifying the source

---

Box 2.1 ▪ Alternative terms for futility[5]

Medical futility
Nonbeneficial treatment
Not clinically appropriate
Not medically indicated
Clinical futility
Medically inappropriate
Medically inadvisable
Potentially inappropriate

of the judgment and possibly implying that treatment might not be futile in a different, nonmedical, sense. Others admit of uncertainty or contextual variation ('potentially inappropriate'). At the end of the day, though, it does not matter what word we use. The ethically important question is: what does it mean?

'Pointless'

Justice Francis, in his first ruling on Charlie Gard, identified what he understood by 'futile'. He described futile treatment as 'pointless, or of no effective benefit'.[6]

This seems very close to a common sense use of the word. If the underground train is on its way out of the station, it would be futile to run after it. If you have a large ink stain from a leaking pen on your shirt, it would be futile to scrub at it with water under the tap. If a patient has been decapitated, it would be futile to attempt to save their life by compressing their chest. These are efforts or actions that have zero chance of achieving their goal. They cannot work.

Of course, even when we know that doing something would be futile, we still sometimes do it – perhaps out of frustration, or desperation or a need to do *something*. But we know in our hearts that it won't do any good.

One thing to notice about defining futile treatment in terms of it being 'pointless' is that it is necessary to be clear, and to agree, on what the 'point' of treatment is. Imagine, for example, that parents bring their 6-year-old child to the doctor during an influenza outbreak with what appears to be influenza. Perhaps the doctor has even performed a new rapid molecular test and confirmed that this is an influenza infection. Imagine now that the parents have requested antibiotics for their son. The doctor might reasonably refuse, regarding it as pointless since viruses do not respond to antibiotics and there is zero chance that the antibiotics will cure influenza. (Giving antibiotics for a viral infection is sometimes suggested as a clear example of a futile treatment.)

However, that may not be why the parents want the antibiotics. They might want them to reduce the chance of developing a secondary bacterial pneumonia; perhaps they have read a scientific paper describing the use of antibiotics in influenza in children and reporting a lower incidence of pneumonia.[7] Or perhaps they had another child become seriously unwell after a previous influenza infection and want to do anything possible to avoid this occurring. If either of those reasons are the point of treatment, it isn't so clear that antibiotics would be futile. They may be unlikely to work. It may be unwise for the doctor to prescribe them (as this would contribute to wider problems of antibiotic resistance). But it isn't clear that it would be futile. After all, children do, rarely, die of secondary bacterial pneumonia after viral flu infections. The antibiotics might prevent that.

Of perhaps more relevance to decisions about life-prolonging treatment, it is sometimes said to be futile to prolong life using a ventilator or other medical treatment for patients who are permanently unconscious. (We will leave aside, for now, the problem of determining someone's level of consciousness or predicting that they will remain so.) That was one of the situations we mentioned earlier that had been identified by Lawrence Scheiderman as being futile. In the highly influential UK court case relating to Tony Bland (a young man who suffered severe brain damage and was left in a persistent vegetative state after being crushed in a football stadium accident), Lord Goff wrote:

> '*I cannot see that medical treatment is appropriate or requisite simply to prolong a patient's life when such treatment has no therapeutic purpose of any kind, as where it is futile because the patient is unconscious and there is no prospect of any improvement in his condition.*'[8]

Many people might share Lord Goff's view. Yet, not everyone will feel that way. In December 2013, a Californian teenage girl, Jahi McMath, suffered a serious life-threatening complication after relatively minor throat surgery. She was resuscitated but sustained profound brain damage. Three days later, Jahi was diagnosed as being brain dead by her physicians, but the family disagreed. They argued that, according to their religious views, she was still alive because her heart was still beating. A Californian court supported the medical diagnosis of death, but the family continued to object to discontinuation of life support. They found a medical facility prepared to take over Jahi's care.[9] As of late 2017, Jahi's body continues to be supported by a mechanical ventilator in New Jersey.[10]

Many health professionals would regard continued mechanical ventilation for a child who has met brain death criteria as paradigmatically, unquestionably, futile. This is surely the ultimate in futile treatment?

If the point of continuing treatment is to cure the patient, then prolonging life with a ventilator would be futile for someone like Jahi McMath because it could not fix her brain damage. If it is truly the case that a patient's condition is permanent, it would be futile to continue treatment in the hope that they will improve (and regain consciousness for example). But Jahi McMath's family wanted treatment continued because they believed that her heart beating meant that she continued to live. Of course, this is no longer the standard of life and death: today, a brain death definition of death is widely accepted in medicine. However, it used to be a cardiorespiratory definition, and based on that definition, she would not be dead. Which definition of death we accept is an ethical decision.[a]

We cannot say that it is pointless to continue medical treatments for Jahi McMath unless there is agreement about what the point of treatment is. We are not defending continued treatment for patients who have been diagnosed as being brain dead. (There are a range of reasons not to continue treatment – most importantly, perhaps, resource concerns (see Chapter 4)). Our argument is simply that, even in cases like this, there can be different views about what the aim of medical treatment is and what constitutes a successful outcome. These can involve contested value judgments. If treatment is going to be refused, that has to be on the basis of a value judgment about what are the appropriate goals of treatment.

The value of zero

If we could identify treatments that have literally no point or no chance of working, there are some ethical advantages.

One advantage is that it potentially neutralises concern about paternalism. Doctors do not always know best, for the principle reason that people differ in what is important to them and how they evaluate medical treatments. What may be right for one person is not right for another. At the heart of disagreements about medical treatment – like that relating to Charlie Gard – are differences in the values that families and professionals place on different options. It may not be clear that one valuation is right and one is wrong. However, accepting that there can be different reasonable ways of evaluating situations or medical treatments does not mean that any evaluation is equally valid. (For more on pluralism, and the difference between pluralism and relativism, see Chapter 7.) There are some evaluations that do appear to be mistaken. The most obvious of these

---

[a]The brain death definition was introduced by a Committee of Harvard Medical school in 1968 to supplement the cardiorespiratory definition for two ethical reasons. Firstly, artificial ventilation and intensive care became very effective, meaning that people could be kept alive for long periods of time even when their brain is irreversibly and catastrophically damaged. Secondly, organ transplantation became feasible and an obvious source was organs from people who were brain dead.[11] For these two very pragmatic reasons, the concept of brain death was proposed and subsequently widely (though not universally) accepted.

would be where a patient desires a treatment that has zero chance of benefit, or objectively has no benefit.

The second advantage lies in the way that courts have thought about decisions to withdraw life-prolonging treatment. Doctors are sometimes in situations where continuing medical treatment will prolong life, but stopping treatment will likely lead fairly quickly to the patient's death. In that situation, there may be good reasons not to want to continue treatment. However, there may also be a concern that stopping treatment means effectively that the doctor (or court) is judging that it would be in the patient's interests to die. It may seem that the doctor or judge would be aiming for the patient to die. The first of these seems philosophically puzzling. How could someone have an interest in being dead – when they will (it is usually believed) have no interests? The second is often thought to be legally problematic. Taking actions that aim at a patient's death are often regarded to be illegal. There are different ways to resolve these concerns. One way, though, takes advantage of the perceived zero benefit of treatment. In the Tony Bland case, Lord Goff wrote:

> 'the question is not whether it is in the best interests of the patient that he should die. The question is whether it is in the best interests of the patient that his life should be prolonged by the continuance of this form of treatment.' (p. 868)

This appears to reverse the judgment. It focuses the judge's or doctors' attention on the questionable treatment, rather than on death. If treatment has no benefit, it need not be provided, even if death will ensue after its removal. In fact, the judges in the Bland case and in subsequent cases have gone further. In a more recent case in the Supreme Court, Lady Hale wrote:

> 'If the treatment is not in his best interests, the court will not be able to give its consent on his behalf and it will follow that it will be lawful to withhold or withdraw it. Indeed, _it will follow that it will not be lawful to give it._'[12] (Emphasis added)

This suggests that it would actually be illegal to provide or continue treatment in a situation of zero benefit.

Zero experience, zero benefit

It might be admitted that, in a situation like that of Jahi McMath, there could be a point to providing treatment (to continue the life of her body, or to respect her parents' religious beliefs). But many might be tempted to think that such treatment would be of zero actual benefit to her since she has no longer any capacity for consciousness.

Brain death seems to be the clearest example where this argument applies. In California, as elsewhere in the US, brain death is determined based on lack of function of the whole brain. Jahi McMath had a series of medical tests of her brain stem reflexes. She also had a series of three electrical recordings (electroencephalograms, EEGs) that showed no electrical signals from her brain.[13]

The exact nature of the relationship between brain activity and consciousness is complex and not completely understood. However, it is clear that brain activity is necessary for consciousness. Without brain function, it does not seem to be conceivable that Jahi has any ability to experience anything – either pain or pleasure. If we assume that conscious experience is the basis for having interests, the corollary in the UK legal system appears to be that treatment would not be in Jahi's interests, and consequently could not be legally continued.

There is, in fact, one UK legal case where parents have requested continued intensive medical treatment in just this sort of situation. In early 2015, a child (named in the court judgment as

'Child A') suffered a cardiac arrest after choking on a small piece of fruit.[14] Child A sustained severe hypoxic brain damage, and 4 days after being admitted to hospital, he was diagnosed as being brain dead. Like in the McMath case, Child A's parents could not accept that he had died – partly because of their religious beliefs. They came originally from Saudi Arabia, where they believed that intensive care would not be withdrawn in such circumstances.[b] They had requested that their son be transferred to Saudi Arabia for continued treatment. The judge in this case did not allow the parents' request and allowed the ventilator to be turned off. This would be consistent with the line of argument alluded to earlier. In actual fact, there was no mention of the interests of Child A in the judgment at all. He was regarded as having died, so perhaps there was or could be no question of interests.[c]

The more common situation, where there is a question about continuing treatment and it might be thought that the patient has no conscious experience (and hence no benefit from treatment), is that of a persistent vegetative state. That was the diagnosis in Tony Bland's case. Lord Browne-Wilkinson in the Bland case wrote: 'The distressing truth which must not be shirked is that is that the proposed conduct is not in the best interests of Anthony Bland, for he has no best interests of any kind.'[17] (Emphasis added)

While this analysis may have been appropriate for Tony Bland, and reflected medical understanding of the vegetative state in 1993, the picture is now more complicated and less clear.[18] Recent advances in neuroscience have suggested that some patients diagnosed with persistent vegetative state (potentially only a minority) retain a limited capacity for consciousness – apparently evidenced by their ability to respond to commands in a way that can be detected by functional neuroimaging or EEG.[19] The implications of this for decisions about life-sustaining treatment are complex.[20] However, one implication is that it is more difficult to rule out consciousness and interests in patients who have been diagnosed as being in a vegetative state.

If a patient definitely has no conscious experience, it might be possible to argue that they have no interests. In the Charlie Gard case, however, it was not argued that he was permanently unconscious. In the High Court case in April, one of the experts at Great Ormond Street testified that the medical team believed that he was 'suffering', implying some level of awareness of his surroundings. (Later in the case in July, a statement from the hospital indicated: 'His depletive genetic disorder leaves him … so far as can be discerned after many months of encephalopathy, without any awareness.'[21] Importantly, if he was 'without any awareness', he could not suffer, and a trial of therapy would not impose any suffering.)

Nearly zero

We could imagine some situations that might truly fit into the category of having no benefit. Some writers have distinguished treatment that would be 'physiologically futile' – that is, where it would be impossible to achieve the intended physiological goal.[2] Physiological goals

---

[b]Diagnosis of brain death, withdrawal of mechanical ventilation and donation of organs are permitted in Saudi Arabia, albeit the criteria are different (and stricter than in the UK).[15] It is not clear, however, whether it is an option to continue mechanical ventilation if families do not accept the diagnosis of death.

[c]Of note, the judge in this case made a concluding comment that ventilation should be withdrawn 'to allow Child A, who died on 10th February, dignity in death'. In the court hearing, Justice Hayden is reported to have said: 'To speak in terms of best interest therefore is redundant, but to respect his young and short life, his dignity, his autonomy, requires me … to do the right thing.'[16] 'Dignity' is an even vaguer and more value-laden concept than 'futility'. We will return in the next chapter to concepts of dignity in death; however, it appears contradictory to hold that someone who is in a vegetative state or brain dead has 'no interests', but then also to claim that they have an interest in 'dignity' or a particular way of being treated.

include, for example, restoration of circulation, remission of cancer or cure of bacterial infection. Yet, the clarity of this form of futility comes at the cost of applicability – it applies to very few of the actual cases where treatment is disputed. Some examples that have been cited of treatment that is physiologically futile include cardiopulmonary resuscitation in a patient who has been decapitated or who has signs of rigor mortis, indicating that they died hours previously. However, neither of these examples are ever likely to yield serious disputes about treatment.

But maybe the chance does not have to be actually zero? You might have noticed Justice Francis' qualifications in his definition of futility in the Gard case.

The judge noted that treatment might be labelled futile if it had 'no *effective* benefit', or if the 'prospect of … benefit is *as close to zero as makes no difference*' [emphasis added]. This seems to allow that treatment could still be called futile if it had some small benefit (but very low in magnitude) or a non-zero (but very small) chance of benefit. This sort of qualification is necessary because, as we alluded to earlier, there are some conceivable benefits of continuing treatment even in cases where most would consider this to be pointless. It is also extremely difficult to prove that there is literally no chance of treatment working. However, as soon as it is admitted that there could be some benefit of treatment, or some chance of treatment working, we then need to engage in an ethical weighing up of those benefits against the negatives of treatment. We will return to that sort of balancing process in the next chapter. For now, though, it is enough to point out that it is necessary to decide how small a benefit is so small that it is not worth pursuing, or how small a chance of treatment would qualify for regarding a treatment as futile. One in a hundred? One in a thousand? One in a million? The difficulty in answering that in clear and coherent way is one of the main reasons why many ethicists have abandoned the concept of futility.

Levels of futility

When the Court of Appeal considered Charlie's case in May, one of the arguments that they considered was whether the High Court had used the wrong definition of futility. There was a distinction between a higher medical concept of futility and a more stringent legal definition that might apply in a smaller number of cases. In a previous case of disputed treatment (for a 68-year-old man, David James, who had a prolonged stay in intensive care after surgery for colon cancer), different definitions of futile treatment had been used by different levels of the court. Doctors had sought permission not to provide intensive support of Mr James' circulation or kidneys or to provide cardiopulmonary resuscitation. There were different views about whether this treatment should be regarded as futile. In the case of Mr James, Sir Alan Ward in the Court of Appeal identified that a core goal of medical treatments is a 'real prospect of curing or at least palliating the life-threatening disease or illness from which the patient is suffering'.[22] He felt that further intensive treatment or resuscitation would be futile because it could not alleviate Mr James' underlying illness. In doing so, he reached a different conclusion from the lower court judge, Judge Peter Jackson, who had evaluated whether the treatment would be 'ineffective or … of no benefit to the patient'. This was a more restrictive test, and the judge had rejected the doctors' request to withhold further treatment; he was not convinced that there was no chance of recovery. Finally, Baroness Hale, in the Supreme Court, concluded that the more stringent test was the correct legal definition: treatments could be of benefit even if they could not cure or alleviate an underlying disease or disability. However, the judge noted that, by the time that the Court of Appeal considered this case, Mr James' medical condition had deteriorated to such a degree that the more strict definition of futility applied.

In the Charlie Gard appeal, the judge felt that these different levels of futility were not relevant as treatment had been identified as futile even on the more strict legal definition.

Proving zero

Even if it were possible to agree on a particular standard for futility, there is a further challenge in assessing whether or not it has been reached for a particular patient. There are several factors contributing to this problem.

One problem is the difficulty in establishing that a treatment has no chance or no benefit. In the Gard judgment, there was considerable mention of the lack of evidence:

> '(20) There is <u>no evidence</u> that nucleoside therapy can cross the blood/brain barrier ...
> (101) [Dr Hirano] confirmed ... that there was <u>no clinical evidence</u> to support the theory ...
> there was no direct evidence that nucleoside therapy has had any beneficial effect on the brain
> (106) The long and the short of Dr I's evidence is that there is <u>no scientific evidence</u> of any
> prospect of any improvement in a human'.

However, it is often observed in medicine that we should distinguish 'absence of evidence' from 'evidence of absence'. There was no direct or clinical evidence presented in the trial that nucleoside therapy would work. But there was no evidence that it would not work either. That was quite simply because it had never been tried.

The point is not that untested treatments can or should necessarily be allowed in children in the absence of evidence. The point is rather that we cannot say that such treatments are futile if we do not know if they will work.

Here is one example that might be relevant:

In 1941, some scientists in Oxford tested a new treatment on a 43-year-old policeman with a serious skin infection. That treatment had never before been tried in a human patient with sepsis. It had been tried in an animal model of a different sort of infection. Patients with this condition usually died, and none of the proven treatments had worked for him. Was it futile to try the new treatment?

Of course, Howard Florey and Charles Fletcher did not know if penicillin would work. It was uncertain if the antibiotic would help, and possible that it would do more harm than good. However, it would have clearly been a mistake to say in advance that treatment with penicillin was futile because there was no direct or clinical evidence of benefit.[23] (Ironically, the penicillin injections administered to Oxford policeman Albert Alexander were ultimately without benefit as he succumbed to his infection after the supply of penicillin ran out. However, the temporary improvement in Albert Alexander and the improvement in other patients where the new treatment was tried led to the widespread use of penicillin and further antibiotics, and to the saving of countless hundreds of millions lives.)

One of the significant contemporary challenges for identifying further treatment as being futile is the ever-expanding number of possible treatments. Of course, there has always been scientific research into new treatments and hope that these might alleviate previously untreatable conditions. What has definitely changed, however, is access to information about those novel therapies. As in the Gard case, parents may search the internet and identify therapies that have been suggested or hypothesised to work, with which their doctors are unfamiliar. There may be the possibility (to a far greater degree than previously) for patients to travel to access those treatments.

What if treatments have been tried before? Can we say then that they won't work? As noted earlier, Schneiderman proposed that treatments could be called futile if they had not worked in 100 previous patients. However, even that evidence would not tell us that treatment could not work in the 101st. All we could say is that the probability of treatment working is low. Statistical models imply that, if something has not been observed in a group of 'n' patients, the 95% confidence interval for the prevalence of this event is between 0 and $\frac{3}{n}$. In other words, if 100 patients have not responded to treatment, we can be reasonably confident that the actual proportion of patients in whom the treatment works is 3% or less.

Next, even if treatment has not worked in past patients, there is a challenge in working out whether or not that can be extrapolated to the current patient. It is challenging to define which group of patients should be used to determine the probability of treatment success. Imagine a patient with advanced cancer who has not responded to treatment, and for whom a new drug is being considered. Should we look at data from all patients who have received the new drug, or only patients with the same type of cancer who have received that drug or only patients of a similar age/general health and type of cancer who have received the drug? The goal of precision medicine is to create very small classes of precisely characterised patients. But there may be multiple different groups of patients at whom we could look, yielding multiple different probabilities. Furthermore, there is an inherent tension between robustness and relevance of our estimates (this is a form of what is called the 'bias-variance trade-off' in statistics). Large case series will usually contain patients with a wide range of different features. Estimates may have small confidence intervals (because they are based on large numbers) but yield potentially biased predictions. On the other hand, there may be little or no published evidence relating to other patients with exactly the same features as the current patient, yielding high variance (very uncertain) predictions. In Charlie Gard's case, there were around five patients in the world with his condition, and none had been treated with nucleoside replacement therapy. Any trial of therapy for such a condition would inevitably involve great uncertainty.

There is a further problem, in that available data on which to base predictions may be affected by the problem of self-fulfilling prophecies.[24] If patients with a given condition are perceived to have a poor prognosis, they may not receive treatment, or treatment may be withdrawn. Subsequently, it can be difficult to know whether the high death rate in that group of patients is because treatment is not provided or because of their underlying condition. That can be a particular problem for predictions in intensive care.

Sometimes, it seems as though some of these difficulties with medical uncertainty are just because of a lack of scientific evidence. They will get easier with time. For example, we now have large amounts of evidence about the use of penicillin or other antibiotics in patients with skin infections. We can use that information to work out whether treatment is likely to work for patients with a particular type of skin infection. We might be tempted to hope that the revolution in medicine with genomic information and personalised medicine will make it easier to make difficult decisions, for example about Child A, Jahi McMath, David James or Charlie Gard. However, there is some reason to think that the problem of applying past evidence to current cases will become an even greater challenge as genomic testing becomes more common. If there is information about a child's specific genetic form of disease, it may become much harder to know whether information from children with other genetic profiles can be applied. In Charlie's case, doctors had evidence from caring for other children with severe mitochondrial disease. There was also evidence from other children with MDDS. However, there was almost no evidence from other children with Charlie's specific genetic form of the disease, RRMB2-related, because it was so rare.

The more specific and the more detailed genomic evidence that becomes available, the harder it will be to apply evidence from other patients. But also, the harder it will be to conclude that treatment cannot work. We will consider some of the challenges in obtaining and interpreting scientific evidence in Chapter 5.

Conclusion

One potential way to resolve disagreements about medical treatment between families and health professionals would be to resort to the concept of futility. However, hoping that futility will make disagreements easy to resolve seems naïve and doomed to fail. The only clear definition of futile treatment on which there appears to be agreement is that of physiologically futile treatment, where there is no physiological mechanism by which treatment could work, and hence no chance of benefit. However, this definition does not appear to apply to the cases that actually come to the courts – like that of Charlie Gard or David James.

In almost all cases where there is a dispute about treatment, there is some chance or some degree of benefit. The real question is whether there is benefit enough to provide it. But to work out whether that is the case, we need to consider the reasons in favour of treatment and the reasons against.

In fact, when we are thinking about disputes about medical treatment for children, there are two important reasons that might justify not providing treatment. Even if there is some possible benefit, treatment should not be provided if overall it would be harmful to the child. Alternatively, even if it wouldn't be harmful to the child, treatment should not be provided if it would harm others (for example, by preventing them from receiving treatment and violating principles of distributive justice). We will consider these separately. First, when would providing treatment be against the child's best interests?

References

1. Schneiderman, L. J., Jecker, N. S. & Jonsen, A. R. (1990) Medical futility: its meaning and ethical implications. *Ann Intern Med*, 112, 949-54.
2. Truog, R. D., Brett, A. S. & Frader, J. (1992) The problem with futility. *N Engl J Med*, 326, 1560-4.
3. Brody, B. A. & Halevy, A. (1995) Is futility a futile concept? *J Med Philos*, 20, 123-44.
4. Helft, P. R., Siegler, M. & Lantos, J. (2000) The rise and fall of the futility movement. *N Engl J Med*, 343, 293-6.
5. Wilkinson, D. J. C. & Savulescu, J. (2011) Knowing when to stop: futility in the ICU. *Curr Opin Anaesthesiol*, 24, 160-5.
6. Great Ormond Street Hospital vs Yates & Ors [2017] EWHC 972 (Fam) (11 April 2017) *para 93.*
7. Maeda, S., Yamada, Y., Nakamura, H. & Maeda, T. (1999) Efficacy of antibiotics against influenza-like illness in an influenza epidemic. *Pediatr Int*, 41, 274-6.
8. *Airedale NHS Trust v Bland* [1993] AC 789.
9. Luce, J. M. (2015) The uncommon case of Jahi McMath. *Chest*, 147, 1144-1151.
10. http://medicalfutility.blogspot.co.uk/2015/10/california-court-allows-jahi-mcmath-to.html
11. (1968) A definition of irreversible coma. Report of the Ad Hoc Committee of the Harvard Medical School to Examine the Definition of Brain Death. *JAMA*, 205, 337-40.
12. *Aintree University Hospital NHS Foundation Trust v. James* [2013] UKSC 67.
13. http://thaddeuspope.com/images/CHO_-_Physician_Decls.pdf.
14. *Re A (A Child)* [2015] EWHC 443 (Fam).
15. http://www.scot.gov.sa/uploads/OPTO/english.pdf.
16. http://www.mirror.co.uk/news/uk-news/its-right-right-thing-do-5171272.
17. *Airedale NHS Trust v Bland. Op cit.*
18. Celesia, G. (2016) Vegetative state two decades after the multi-society task force (MSTF) Report. in M. M. Monti and W. Sannita (Eds.) *Brain function and responsiveness in disorders of consciousness.* Cham, Springer.
19. Monti, M. M., Vanhaudenhuyse, A., Coleman, M. R., Boly, M., Pickard, J. D., Tshibanda, L., et al. (2010) Willful modulation of brain activity in disorders of consciousness. *N Engl J Med*, 362, 579-89.
20. Skene, L., Wilkinson, D., Kahane, G. & Savulescu, J. (2009) Neuroimaging and the withdrawal of life-sustaining treatment from patients in vegetative state. *Med Law Rev*, 17, 245-61.
21. *GOSH position statement to the court 13 July* http://thaddeuspope.com/images/Great_Ormond_Street_Hospital_Position_Statement_UK_High_Court_13_July_2017_pdf
22. *Aintree University Hospital NHS Foundation Trust v. James* Op cit.
23. Greenwood, D. (2008) *Antimicrobial drugs : chronicle of a twentieth century medical triumph.* Oxford, Oxford University Press.
24. Wilkinson, D. (2009) The self-fulfilling prophecy in intensive care. *Theoretical medicine and bioethics*, 30, 401-10.

CHAPTER 3

Best interests

"If any one of them can explain it," said Alice ... "I'll give him sixpence.
I don't believe there's an atom of meaning in it."
"If there's no meaning in it," said the King, "that saves a world of trouble,
you know, as we needn't try to find any. And yet I don't know," he went on,
spreading out the verse on his knee, and looking at them with one eye; "I seem
to see some meaning in them, after all."'

Alice's Adventures in Wonderland, Lewis Carroll

'*the intellectual milestones for the judge in a case such as the present are, therefore, simple, although the ultimate decision will frequently be extremely difficult. The judge must decide what is in the child's best interests. In making that decision, the welfare of the child is paramount, ... The term "best interests" encompasses medical, emotional, and all other welfare issues.*'

WYATT V. PORTSMOUTH NHS TRUST [2000] 1 FLR 554
(QUOTED BY JUSTICE FRANCIS IN CHARLIE GARD JUDGMENT).

'*the only course now in Charlie's best interests is to let him slip away peacefully and not put him through more pain and suffering.*'

JUSTICE FRANCIS, HIGH COURT, 11 APRIL. 128

'*it is said, firstly, that the judge ... gave undue weight to the possibility of pain and suffering.*'

JUSTICE MACFARLANE, COURT OF APPEAL – CITING GROUNDS FOR
APPEALING AGAINST HIGH COURT ASSESSMENT OF CHARLIE GARD'S BEST INTERESTS.

In the previous chapter, we argued that it is rare that continuing life-sustaining treatment would have absolutely zero benefit. Instead, there is usually a need to weigh up, or balance, the possible benefits against the possible harms of treatment.

The metaphor of 'balancing' the positives and negatives of providing treatment has sometimes been taken quite literally. In some cases of disputed treatment, the UK courts have asked legal teams to draw up a 'balance sheet', with the reasons in favour of treatment on one side of the page, and the reasons against on the other.

While it might be more controversial to list the pros and cons of life versus death, this sort of assessment is, in fact, no different from the sort of process that we all go through when we are deciding about any medical treatment (or indeed for many other major decisions in life). Are the pain, disruption and risks of having a knee replacement worth it to be able to walk or exercise more easily and without discomfort? Are the potential side effects and inconvenience of taking drugs every day worth it to reduce the risk of a heart attack? A lot of the time, the positives will outweigh the negatives, and it will be worth undergoing surgery or taking medicines. Sometimes, though, the scales are tipped the other way.

When could it not be in a child's best interests to prolong their life? Thinking of the balancing metaphor – this could happen if there is less weight on the positive side of the scales – a child would benefit less from continued treatment. Alternatively, it could happen if the burden side of the scales is weightier – principally, where a child would suffer from treatment. Or, both could happen. There might be situations where there are both fewer reasons in favour of treatment and more reasons against (Fig. 3.1).

In this chapter, we will scrutinise some of the different reasons that apply to prolonging life with medical treatment. We identify different views about when these reasons would count against treatment and the challenge that creates for resolving disagreement. We will see that some reasons provide a stronger or clearer basis for discontinuing treatment, while others are more subject to reasonable disagreement.

Different reasons

What reasons could be given for thinking that life-sustaining treatment is not in a child's best interests? One simple taxonomy or classification system is provided in a guideline for health professionals published by the UK Royal College of Paediatrics and Child Health (RCPCH) in 2015.[1] It identifies two groups of reasons, each of which contains three subcategories (Table 3.1).

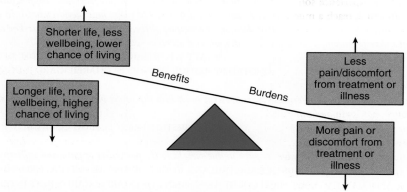

Fig. 3.1 Weighing up a child's best interests. The positives (benefits) of treatment and continued life are on the left scale of the scale, while the negatives are on the right.

TABLE 3.1 ■ **Ethical reasons to limit or forego treatment that could prolong life**

Limited quantity of life	
Brain death	A child has irreversibly lost their capacity for consciousness and their capacity to breathe, and fulfils neurological criteria for death.
Imminent death	A child is physiologically deteriorating and expected to die within minutes or hours.
Inevitable death	A child is expected to die despite treatment (e.g., within a period of days or weeks).
Limited quality of life	
Burdens of treatment	Life can only be sustained at the cost of significant pain or distress.
Burdens of illness or underlying condition	The severity or impact of an underlying condition causes pain and distress that would outweigh the benefits of sustaining life.
Lack of ability to derive benefit	The nature or severity of a child's underlying condition makes it difficult or impossible for them to enjoy the benefits of continued life.

We will consider some of these reasons separately. In addition, we will look at two reasons that aren't described in the RCPCH framework, but that have been cited in cases of disputes: reduced probability of benefit and dignity in dying.

Reduced quantity of life

If treatment could prolong life, but only for a limited amount of time, that might reduce the benefit side of the scales and count against life-prolonging treatment.

The most extreme example of this is where the individual is already regarded as deceased, in which case they have zero life ahead of them.[a] As noted in the previous chapter, such individuals appear to be the clearest example where there is zero benefit from treatment. At the other extreme, children may have a reduced life expectancy as a result of an underlying illness (for example a severe genetic disorder) but could survive into later childhood or early adulthood.

The shorter a child's future life, the less reason there is to provide life-prolonging treatment. Where a patient would survive for a longer time, it may be unclear whether providing a treatment like intensive care would be an overall benefit. That will depend on how unpleasant treatment would be, as well as on how much the child would be able to enjoy their remaining time. We can imagine situations where prolonging an adult's life for even a short period could be important to allow them to experience something that has particular meaning or importance (perhaps to see a new grandchild, reach a milestone birthday or wrap up personal affairs). Those sort of reasons, however, are not going to be relevant to a very young child or to an older child who has limited awareness.

On the other hand, where a child is only going to survive for a short period, that may also reduce the badness of providing unpleasant treatment. Short periods of suffering may not be good, but at least they are short.

One situation where this is particularly relevant is in relation to provision of cardiopulmonary resuscitation (CPR) for seriously ill children. Doctors and nurses sometimes do not want to provide CPR for a child who is gravely ill because they believe that the development of a slow or absent heart beat (which in other situations would prompt doctors to start compressing the chest in an attempt to revive the child) is actually a sign of the child imminently dying.

For example, a few years ago, one of us cared for a newborn infant, 'Jan', with a rare genetic condition that made his heart muscle weak and caused it to fail.[b] Unfortunately, there was no option of heart transplantation, and he had deteriorated despite all available medical treatments. He was on a breathing machine and becoming sicker each day. It was expected that at some point his heart would no longer be able to continue, and would slow and stop. The medical team explained to his family this situation, and that they believed that he was dying. Jan's parents, though, found it difficult to accept the news and did not agree with the doctors that it would be best not to attempt to resuscitate Jan in the event of his heart stopping. They wanted 'everything' to be done to save Jan.

In a case like Jan's, where the quantity of life remaining for the child is so small, it might not be in the child's interests to resuscitate them. However, if a child will die in any case, particularly if they are thought to be 'beyond suffering', there may also appear to be little downside to providing CPR. For example, US intensive care paediatrician and ethicist Robert Truog has argued that it would be justified to provide CPR in just these circumstances – for the sake of the family.[3] In

---

[a]'Life-prolonging treatment' would appear to be a misnomer if a patient is already deceased. Some regard patients who fulfil neurological criteria for death as being alive but profoundly disabled.[2] In that case, this would actually fall within the 'quality of life' category.
[b]This is a composite version of several cases encountered by DW.

reply, ethicist John Paris and colleagues have argued that a compassionate response to Jan and his family would not include providing CPR if his heart stopped. The doctors should examine him, declare him dead and assure the family that 'everything possible' had been done to help him.[4]

Dignity in death

One argument against providing treatments like CPR that would prolong life for only a very short time (if at all) is that this would compromise the child's dignity. In the Charlie Gard case, doctors at Great Ormond Street testified that they believed that 'he should be allowed to die peacefully and with dignity', while Justice Francis ruled that treatment should be withdrawn 'to permit Charlie to die with dignity'.[5]

In the earlier case of Child A (who had been diagnosed as brain dead), Justice Hayden decided that:

> 'the time has now come to permit the ventilator to be turned off and to allow Child A, who died on 10th February, dignity in death'.[6]

In the last chapter, we discussed the case of Mr James, who was deteriorating after a prolonged intensive care stay. When judges were considering treatment for him, they noted that 'where the patient is close to death, the object may properly be to make his dying as comfortable and as dignified as possible, rather than to take invasive steps to prolong his life for a short while'.[7]

However, it is unclear in these legal cases, and others, what exactly is meant by 'dignity' in death, or what ethical significance this should have. One possibility is that a dignified death refers to dying in a place and time of one's choosing. In debates about assisted dying, advocates for 'dying with dignity' often seem to have this sort of idea in mind. However, this could not apply to cases relating to children like Child A or Charlie Gard, who have never made such a choice. It also could not apply to Mr James as his family denied that he would have wanted intensive care to be limited in the way that doctors planned. Another possible meaning would be that dying while receiving treatments that are causing suffering (out of proportion to benefit) would be undignified. Yet that interpretation would imply that the concept of dignity could be reduced to the question of best interests – it is the same thing, except by a different name. It also would not make any sense in relation to Child A, who clearly was not suffering (and had already died).

The most obvious way of understanding the concept of dignity as used in these cases is that there are particular ways of dying and particular ways of treating those who are deceased that are 'dignified'. It seems that judges and doctors have in mind that a death that is peaceful, free from pain and medical intervention is quintessentially dignified, while a death that is accompanied by pain or by particularly invasive or intrusive medical interventions is not dignified. In the case of a child with severe hypoxic brain injury (as well as underlying physical disability), Justice Macdonald made this clear:

> 'when it is recognised that life is ending, for many the concept of dignity becomes encapsulated by the idea of a "peaceful" or "good" death.'[8]

When it comes to treatment of patients who have died (or perhaps are in the last phase of dying), there is an intuitive sense that it is important to treat them with respect or dignity, even if they could never be aware of how they are treated. If you have ever read media reports of soldiers who have mutilated or paraded the dead bodies of their enemies, you might share the view that this shows a profound lack of respect for the deceased and represents an additional wrong or harm inflicted on the enemy soldiers.

However, if there is an objective sense of dignity here, we should note that there are some very different (and contradictory) views about what would count as dignified treatment at the end of life.[c] While some would doubtless feel strongly that a peaceful death, free from medical intervention, is dignified, there are others who see dignity in struggle and resistance. They may share the sentiment of Welsh poet Dylan Thomas: 'Do not go gentle into that good night, old age should burn and rave at close of day'.[9] Philosopher Frances Kamm has pointed out that peacefulness in death might not always be desired or fit with someone's core beliefs (e.g., if someone believed that they would be punished after death).[10]

We will discuss in Chapter 4 the case of Jaymee Bowen. There was disagreement about whether she should receive a second bone marrow transplant for relapsed leukaemia. Her doctors initially argued that a second transplant was not in her best interests. Jaymee was interviewed later as an 11-year-old (after receiving the transplant privately) for a television documentary. Her advice to other children in her position echoes Dylan Thomas: 'Never give up. Never give up until you are on the last little drop of life.'[11]

It may be that most people regard it as undignified to continue mechanical ventilation in a patient who meets criteria for brain death. However, that clearly wasn't the view of Child A's parents, nor does it appear to be the view of the parents of the brain dead teenager Jahi McMath. One of the difficulties with this argument against treatment (that treatment would lead to an undignified death) is that there is no obvious way to arbitrate between some very different views about dignity at the end of life. Another is that, despite its widespread usage in end-of-life debates, it is rarely, if ever, formally defined. It could be argued that dignity serves as a way of prematurely foreclosing debate, or of imposing on others a particular view about what kind of death is desirable.

Reduced quality of life

The phenomenon of diverging views about a key ethical question, highlighted in relation to the concept of dignity in death, might apply even more forcefully to the question of quality of life. Table 3.1 separates out reasons for limiting treatment into those based on reduced quantity of life from those based on reduced quality of life. In practice, there is almost always a combination of the two. In almost all cases of disputed treatment that reach the courts, there is reason to believe that the child would suffer from treatment, would suffer from their underlying illness or, even if they are not suffering, would benefit very little.

In fact, in the Charlie Gard case, the question of Charlie's current quality of life was a point of rare apparent agreement. Both his parents and health professionals agreed that his quality of life (he was deaf, paralysed and dependent on a breathing machine in intensive care) was not acceptable and should not be prolonged. His parents told the court: 'We would not fight for the quality of life he has now.' (para 110)

But what about in other cases? How should we evaluate quality of life? In particular, how should we answer the question of whether someone's quality of life is good enough that they should receive life-prolonging medical treatment?

Before we address that question, it is important to note that, whenever there is discussion about whether a life is worth living or worth prolonging, some people worry that this judgment is about the value of an individual to others. In this chapter, though, we are focusing our attention

---

[c]The Ancient Greek historian Herodotus famously described the Persian king Darius's experience of cultural norms around death. Darius summoned some Greeks and asked them whether they would eat their dead fathers. They were horrified at the idea. He was then said to have invited some Indians (whose custom it was to eat their dead parents) to ask them whether they would burn the bodies of their parents. They were horrified. Herodotus commented: 'one can see by this what custom can do'.[12]

on the question of best interests – what would be best for the individual. The question is whether, for that individual, the benefits of treatment outweigh the burdens. It is about the value of that child's life for them.

One example of a serious illness where this quality of life question has been raised is for children with a very severe form of muscle weakness, spinal muscular atrophy. This genetic disorder leads to progressive loss of the nerve supply to the body's muscles. There are different forms, but the most severe form affects newborn infants. As in Charlie Gard's case, infants with this condition often appear healthy at birth, but develop worsening muscle weakness in the early weeks and months of life, eventually progressing to a point where they cannot breathe and need support from a ventilator. When this occurs, doctors will often recommend withdrawal of life support with the expectation that the infant will die.

There have been a number of cases in the UK where parents of children with severe spinal muscular atrophy have disagreed with health professionals about treatment for a child with spinal muscular atrophy, and where those disagreements have reached the court:

1998 'C' – 16-month-old infant. Court authorised withdrawal of mechanical ventilation against the wishes of his parents.

2006 'MB' – 18-month-old child. Court did not authorise withdrawal of treatment – treatment continued.

2015 'Y' – 7-year-old girl with less severe form of spinal muscular atrophy, previously not dependent on a ventilator. Deterioration with development of additional brain damage, now dependent on continuous noninvasive breathing support. Court authorised doctors not to intubate and place Y on a ventilator, and not to resuscitate her in the event of a cardiac arrest.

2016 – 3½-month-old child, on a ventilator since soon after birth. Court authorised withdrawal of treatment.[8,13-15]

For children with the most severe forms of spinal muscular atrophy, they often reach a point where they are completely paralysed, able to control movement of only their eyes or a finger. Unlike in children with Charlie Gard's condition, children with spinal muscular atrophy usually have normal learning and cognitive (thinking) abilities. With provision of long-term breathing support, it can be possible for children with this condition to survive for many years.[16]

In 2013, Australian doctors published the case of Yasmin, an 8-year-old girl with spinal muscular atrophy who had remained in hospital, connected to a breathing machine, since infancy. When Yasmin was first diagnosed, there had been disagreement between doctors and parents, with doctors feeling strongly that it was not in Yasmin's best interests to keep her alive and her parents refusing to allow withdrawal of breathing support.[17] In that case, however, doctors had elected (despite misgivings) to continue treatment. At age 8, several of the health professionals decided to publish some of the details of Yasmin's case in order to promote discussion of the ethics of treatment in such cases.[18] Yasmin remained in hospital in a paediatric ward because her parents felt unable to care for her at home, while no foster family had been able to be found. Kelly Gray, a case coordinator at the hospital described Yasmin's situation:

'Yasmin is mostly a happy child. She is under constant nursing care in a three-bedded room on a ward. Her daily timetable comprises of almost continuous cares including medication, hygiene, nappy changes, repositioning, therapy, charted observations and bracing regimes ... She especially enjoys attending school several days a week. It is possible to discern Yasmin's mood through facial and other physiological signs. She is able to smile (minimally), she can wiggle her index finger and legs, and at times, she vocalises (by tooting around her tracheostomy).

However, there are times when Yasmin is discernibly unhappy. She is unhappy when her parents leave. She becomes upset if her parents cancel a visit. She enjoys outings but dislikes returning to the ward. These are all things we see in cognitively normal children. How do we know what

Yasmin likes and dislikes? While she is unable to cry the way a normal child does, she displays almost all the same signs. Her eyes produce tears and her face becomes red. Her heart rate increases and her oxygen saturation levels decline. But, as she is unable to move or speak, if no one is directly looking at her, she can sometimes become silently distressed.'[18]

Do the benefits of medical treatment outweigh the burdens for Yasmin? Some people would be tempted to answer that this is ultimately subjective.

Is quality of life subjective?

One way that quality of life could be subjective would be if this is something that only the individual (or 'subject') can answer for themselves. For example, we can ask a competent adult about how well their life is going, and whether they would like to be provided with medical treatment to prolong their life. One person might answer that this would be worthwhile, whereas another would not. For adults who are very sick in intensive care, even if we cannot ask them, we could ask close family members or friends about the patient's wishes and values, and whether it is likely that they would judge their current and future quality of life as good enough to prolong with treatment.

But if we can only assess someone's quality of life by asking them, then there is no way to determine quality of life for infants (or children or adults) like Yasmin who cannot express a view about their quality of life. There would be no way to work out whether treatment would be in the child's best interests, and no way of resolving disagreements. Perhaps in that situation we should just rely on parents' view about a child's quality of life?

One reason to ask parents would be based on a different way in which quality of life could be subjective. Some people think that quality of life is relative. It is just a matter of personal opinion. What would be a good quality of life for one person would be unacceptable for someone else. It is all in the eye of the beholder. That sense of quality of life being subjective might support the view that we should rely on people's own view about their quality of life, or parents' view about their children's quality of life. If Yasmin's parents think her quality of life is acceptable, that is all there is to say about it.

There are, though, some uncomfortable implications of this view. If it is just a question of personal opinion, it seems that there would be nothing wrong with a view that it would be good to prolong the life of a child in constant, unremitting agony. If an anorexic patient were competent and desired to continue dieting, that would be the best life for her on this view. Equally, there would be nothing wrong with someone else's view that a child with a minor physical disability would have such a poor quality of life that this should not be prolonged with treatment, even though we expected that they would enjoy a full and rich range of activities. If we think that quality of life is purely relative, we could not object to these views or complain that they are mistaken. But that doesn't seem right.

There is a different way that quality of life could be subjective. When philosophers discuss quality of life, they often refer to the concept of 'wellbeing', i.e., how well a life is going. There are two different broad schools of thought about wellbeing. Subjective views about wellbeing focus on the conscious experiences of the individual or on their desires. On these views, life goes well if the individual has positive (or pleasurable) experiences, and doesn't have unpleasant (e.g., painful) experiences. Alternatively, life goes well if the things that the person desires are fulfilled (for example, if they achieve a long-term goal). These two variations of a subjective view are closely related. Usually people strongly desire pleasurable experiences, while also experiencing pleasure if things that they desire come to fruition.

There are also so-called objective views about wellbeing. On those views, there are some things that make someone's life go well apart from by causing pleasure or being wanted. An objective theory would make sense of the idea that someone could sacrifice pleasure or give up something that they desire (for example, for the sake of a relationship with a partner or parent), and that this would make their life overall a better one. There are different things that might be placed on a list of objective valuable features of human life, but they might include, for example, health, autonomy, knowledge, communication, deep personal relationships, accomplishment and enjoyments and avoidance of pain.[d]

As the contents of this list suggest, objective accounts of wellbeing overlap with subjective accounts in that they typically include things that are desired (autonomy, accomplishments) or enjoyed. Furthermore, the views of individuals about what makes their life go well or badly are going to be highly relevant to what might plausibly go in such a list, or how we should evaluate particular states. As an example, individuals with disabilities often have much more positive evaluations of the quality of their life than other (nondisabled) people would expect or imagine. This is sometimes referred to as the 'disability paradox'.[22] One way of understanding this evidence is to point to the many objectively valuable features of life that remain available, despite severe illness or impairment. For example, someone with severe physical disability could still enjoy deep personal relationships, communication, knowledge, accomplishment and autonomy.

On subjective views about wellbeing, it is very important to know what people's views are about how well their life is going. It is, obviously, highly relevant to know how much pain or discomfort they are experiencing, as well as how much pleasure. It is vital to know what the individual's desires are – about medical treatment and about other important things in their life. However, if we are thinking about quality of life in this way, we should be clear that it isn't simply a matter of personal opinion.

Imagine that there is a choice between two different medical treatments for a child that are equally effective, but one of which is much more painful. There isn't any advantage of the more painful treatment. If parents choose for the child to undergo the more painful treatment, there would be strong reason to try to persuade them otherwise. It seems that they are making a mistake. There is a clear sense that their choice will be worse for the child, and there would need to be a very good reason to allow such a choice.[e]

However, as we mentioned already, there is a serious problem with subjective views about quality of life or wellbeing when it comes to patients who cannot communicate. How can we know if they are suffering, or how much they are suffering? How can we know if they have desires, or what they desire or would desire?

Faced with this inability to answer the question, some people might reply that we should just provide or continue life-prolonging medical treatment. Wouldn't that be the safe thing to do? However, dodging the question isn't an option. Providing treatment, and prolonging life in situations where we cannot ask the individual, assumes that treatment is of overall benefit and that life is worth prolonging. It is answering the question – in the affirmative. But we know that, in similar situations, at least some adults would not wish to have their life prolonged with treatment. Quite often, in the cases that reach the courts, the situations are so serious that most adults would not want the treatment that is being requested for a child.[f] There is good reason to think that, at least in some of these cases, providing treatment would be harmful.

---

[d]From the previous section, dignity in dying might be conceived of as an objective value.[19-21]

[e]That does not mean that this option is ruled out. We will consider in Chapter 6 how much weight should be given to the interests of parents. Sometime parents will have a reason for choosing a more painful treatment - perhaps a religious reason. Then the question arises whether that is a sufficiently good reason. (In the case of Jehovah's Witnesses, they believe that if they refuse blood, including blood transfusion, they will go to Heaven. Courts will authorise such treatment for a child. One reason for this is that a parent's religious beliefs are not a good reason to impose harm on a child.)

[f]For example, two-thirds of the general public indicated in a survey that they would wish for life-prolonging medical treatment to be withdrawn if they were in a vegetative state.[23]

If we are to make any sense of decisions about medical treatment for infants, or for older patients whose personal experience and wishes are unknown, we are forced to turn instead to an objective understanding of wellbeing. We cannot determine what exactly they are experiencing. But, nor can we avoid the question.

We argued earlier that thinking about quality of life from a subjective point of view does not mean that quality of life is purely a matter of personal opinion. But if we are thinking about quality of life from an objective viewpoint, we should be careful not to make the opposite mistake. We shouldn't assume that there is a single right answer to what would be in a child's (objective) best interests. We listed some of the potential values that might be included in an objective assessment of wellbeing, and hence, in an objective answer to whether quality of life is good enough to prolong with medical treatment. They included health, autonomy, knowledge, communication, deep personal relationships, accomplishment and enjoyments and avoidance of pain. However, there are two immediate problems. The first is that there is no consensus about what should be included on this list.[24] One alternative list includes moral goodness, rational activity, development of abilities, having children and being a good parent, knowledge and awareness of true beauty.[25] Philosophers disagree about the objective values in human life, and we expect that nonphilosophers, too, might put different things on this list.

The second problem is that with multiple different things on the list, it isn't clear how to combine them. What if someone has richer or deeper personal relationships, but less health or autonomy? How do we weigh up negative values like pain against positives like accomplishment?

Here we face a serious challenge in disagreements about treatment that relate to a child's quality of life. We have argued that we need to think about quality of life in an objective way. However, there can be very different views about whether life would be objectively worth prolonging with medical treatment, either because people see different things as being valuable, or because they give different weights to those valuable features.

There may be some areas of common ground between different views. For example, as noted already, one reason why disability or illness does not necessarily make a life not worth living is because a loss in one area can be compensated in others. If a child's medical condition means that they have severely diminished health and autonomy, but they are still able to have deep personal relationships, communication and enjoyments, that still makes it quite possible that, for them, their life would be worth prolonging. Returning to the metaphor of the set of scales (Fig. 3.1), there would still be important positives on the left side of the scales to be weighed against the negatives. On the other hand, if a child's condition led to a reduction or prevention of many or most of the things in human life that are generally considered valuable, that would mean that there would be very little left on the benefit side of the scales. It would make it much easier for the balance to be tipped, and for the negatives of treatment to outweigh the positives.

There are two important implications of this way of thinking about quality of life and best interests.

TYPES OF DISABILITY

The first implication is about which health conditions are most significant for quality of life. Disabilities are relevant if they reduce the benefits for a child of prolonging life. This is much more likely with conditions that cause severe brain disorders (particularly severe or profound cognitive disability) than with physical conditions and physical disability.[26] Even in the setting of an extremely severe physical disability like spinal muscular atrophy, a child may still be able to benefit from life. In Yasmin's case, it appeared that she recognised and responded to medical professionals and to her family. She seemed to enjoy school and excursions. She had limited ability to communicate and express her desires and was very dependent on others for care.

However, it did appear that she had some benefit from her life.[g] While some of the health professionals caring for Yasmin had different views, it seems in that case that there could be reasonable disagreement about whether it is in her best interests to continue life-prolonging treatment. However, if there was evidence of additional severe cognitive impairment, that might change.

In one of the recent cases that came to the UK court, an 8-year-old girl with spinal muscular atrophy, 'Y', had (before a recent illness) been profoundly physically disabled, but was felt to have a good quality of life. She was not able to sit or stand and needed breathing support overnight. However, she was 'alert, smiling and interactive', and 'had previously been verbally communicative and had made use of an iPad'. Later, though, she had suffered two episodes of out-of-hospital cardiorespiratory arrest, and as a result had sustained severe brain damage from lack of oxygen. One of the specialists in that case gave evidence that Y 'now made no attempt at communication and showed no evidence of cognitive activity. He considered that she no longer made any purposeful movement, that she was unable to communicate and that she was unable to fix and follow'.[8]

This case makes clear the relevance of taking an objective view of best interests.

Severe cognitive disability can prevent the child from communicating, from developing or attaining goals, from being autonomous, from gaining knowledge and from (in some cases) appreciating deep personal relationships. In Y's case, it was reasonably clear that, before her deterioration, she had a life worth living. There were sufficient benefits to outweigh the burdens of life-prolonging medical treatment, and it was in her best interests to receive that treatment. However, when she developed additional severe brain damage, that was no longer the case. The scales began to tip against prolonging her life with medical treatment.

SUFFERING

The second important implication of the view that we have sketched above is that, even if the objective benefits are reduced, treatment might still be in a child's best interests if there is little on the negative (right) side of the scales. If a child isn't suffering, and wouldn't suffer with treatment, it might be still in their best interests for life to be prolonged. So far, we have not paid much attention to the negative side of wellbeing. On the face of it, pain or distress from treatment or, despite treatment, from a child's underlying illness seems like a much easier and less controversial factor. We might ultimately think that this is a stronger ethical rationale than a reduction in benefits of treatment. However, as we will see, there are very considerable challenges in some cases in working out how much weight to place on this side of the scales.

Suffering from treatment

One of the central questions in the Charlie Gard case was whether he was suffering or would suffer from continuing life support over a period of months. This question is also relevant in many other disputes about prolonging intensive care. In a case in early 2016 about whether doctors should provide CPR to a 6-month-old infant with severe brain damage, the judge found that:

'The disadvantages were numerous, but primarily that Y would endure great suffering.'[27]

If treatment is burdensome or unpleasant, that provides a powerful reason that needs to be balanced against the benefits of treatment. On the other hand, if the child wouldn't suffer, it might be ethical to provide treatment even where the benefits would be small or unlikely.

---

[g]This may provide additional reason to provide treatment or assistance that would help a physically disabled child to communicate or be independent.

There are some reasons to worry about pain from treatment. Being kept alive in intensive care is not pleasant. Children on long-term ventilation are frequently subjected to invasive procedures. This includes regular blood tests to monitor organ function, as well as insertion of tubing into blood vessels for monitoring or administration of drugs. Patients on ventilators can frequently experience feelings of being unable to breathe.[28] Breathing tubes become filled with secretions that can cause a patient to have difficulty breathing. If they are unable to cough effectively (and most sick patients in intensive care cannot), they will need suctioning – where a tube is passed into their trachea to remove mucous – a procedure that can be painful or cause a sensation of choking. Patients may have life-threatening and potentially terrifying episodes if their breathing tubes become blocked and require urgent replacement. Qualitative research with adults who have been in intensive care reveals that many recalled unpleasant experiences, including fear, anxiety or panic, sleep deprivation, lack of control, nightmares and loneliness.[29-31]

There are a number of challenges, though, in working out whether or how much individual patients are suffering. The first is that patients who are sick and in intensive care are often unable to communicate. They often cannot tell us what they are experiencing. They may have a breathing tube in their mouth and be unable to speak. They may be sedated or too sick to answer questions. (In many of the cases of disputed treatment, children are too young to speak.) In those situations, doctors and nurses rely on indirect signs of distress, facial expressions, tears and elevations in blood pressure or heart rate. Those signs can be helpful, but their absence isn't always reassuring. In Charlie's case, his muscles were so weak that he could not move. In other patients in intensive care, medication or illness may similarly remove or dampen the outward signs of distress. That raises the prospect that such patients may be frightened, stressed or in pain; with no means of communicating it, their distress goes unrelieved. Yasmin's care coordinator described periods of 'silent distress'.[18]

However, there are also several reasons that suffering might not count against continued treatment. The first is that there are medical means of relieving patient discomfort in intensive care. These include pharmacological sedation (making the patient sleepy or unconscious, but without reducing pain) or pain relief (which directly reduces feelings of pain and may or may not make the patient more sleepy). It also includes topical or local anaesthesia, as well as non-pharmacological means (e.g., reassurance, consoling, distraction). For patients who are gravely ill, they may receive heavy doses of medicines that are akin to general anaesthesia. This should, at least in theory, remove any suffering that results from providing intensive care.

In practice, though, treatment of pain and discomfort is often incomplete or imperfect. In the studies mentioned earlier describing patients' experience of intensive care, the patients had been receiving medicines for pain. Pain is common in hospitalised children – despite attempts to relieve or avoid it.[32] One reason why pain control is not perfect is that there can be a trade-off between the benefits and risks of sedation. Heavy sedation may mean that other drugs (to support blood pressure) are needed. It may hamper efforts to assess the patient's brain function, or make it harder to help the patient in other ways (for example, it is much more difficult to reduce support from the ventilator if a patient is heavily sedated). Over a long period, heavy sedation can increase medical complications such as muscle weakness or chest infections. Children or adults also become accustomed to the medicines, so that the dose needs to be increased to keep on top of their pain, or they need to be switched to other drugs. Furthermore, parents or medical professionals may be reluctant for the child to be heavily sedated. Sedation to unconsciousness might avoid pain – but it would also preclude any interaction with the child and reduce the benefit of keeping the child alive.

There is one group of patients where the question of suffering from treatment is very hard to pin down. Where patients have very abnormal brain function, it may be difficult to know whether they are in pain. As already mentioned, they could experience pain but have no ability to display outward signs. Alternatively, they may be so severely affected that they do not even have any awareness. We noted in the last chapter that there was some ambiguity about Charlie Gard's experience of pain. In the last stages of court appeals, the hospital released a statement describing his current state:

> '[as] far as can be discerned after many months of encephalopathy, [he is] without any awareness. At the moment, he is on a low dose of oral morphine. Before that was started quite recently, all of those caring for him at GOSH hoped very much that Charlie did not experience pain. They did so in the knowledge that if he did not, it was because he had no experience at all because he was beyond experience.'[33]

The hospital appeared to be hedging their bets. If Charlie lacked any capacity for awareness, then there was no need for pain relief (and arguably, no reason to oppose the parents' request for treatment to continue). However, if there was real concern for suffering, low dose oral morphine could seem to be insufficient.

In our personal experience (DW), doctors in this situation sometimes find themselves in an uncomfortable compromise. Parents might be opposed to doctors using higher doses of pain relief if they see the drugs as a cause of their child's failure to improve in intensive care (show signs of neurological recovery). So, they may not be able to optimally treat a child's pain. In other cases, doctors might feel able to stop pain relief in a child who is severely encephalopathic, on the basis that the child (probably) is not able to experience pain. However, if they stop pain relief (because they are certain that the patient is not in pain), that would undermine one of the strongest arguments against continuing treatment. So, they might continue low dose pain relief 'just in case' the patient actually can feel pain.

Another final reason to be sceptical about the harm argument is that, while continued treatment in intensive care is not pleasant, there are many children and adults who every day receive the same or similar treatment. We do not worry about treatment for those patients, so why be concerned about a few months of treatment for a child like Charlie? Isn't treatment a problem for those others? One answer is that treatment for those other patients is unpleasant and painful. But it may be worth putting the child through that pain and discomfort if there is a good chance that the child will recover and leave the intensive care unit. However, where that chance is very slim, it is no longer so clear.

Small chances

We have discussed two factors that might influence the left (positive) side of our best interests scales: quantity (length) of life and quality of life. But there may be uncertainty about each of these. We now turn to the influence of probability on the balance. In the previous chapter, we described the difficulty in establishing that there is no chance of a treatment working. But even if it is not zero, perhaps it is (in Justice Francis' terms) 'as close to zero as makes no difference'? How small is too small a chance?

One point worth making is that there may not be a single answer to this question.

When people are faced with the news of a terminal illness, some seize at any treatment that offers them a chance at longer life. Others decide to forego medical treatment and concentrate on the quality of their remaining time, even if medicines could offer a real prospect of improvement.

That is all very well for an adult who can make up their mind about the risks and benefits of treatment. But how about a child? How do we decide what would be in their best interests?

One important consideration is going to be the burden of treatment. Is it painful to administer, are there side effects, are there risks of making the child's condition worse? The more unpleasant the treatment, presumably the higher the chance would need to be that treatment will work.

Conversely, if the treatment is innocuous, it might be in a child's best interests to receive it even if the chance of it working were very small.

In Charlie's case, while the treatment itself (nucleoside therapy) was felt to be benign, the principal concern was that continuing intensive care would cause him to suffer. We have already mentioned the challenge of answering whether or how much Charlie was suffering.

However, one potential view would be that, even if being kept alive on a ventilator were causing Charlie pain and discomfort, it would be a small price to pay if he were actually to improve from nucleoside treatment.

Imagine, for the sake of argument, that there was actually a 1 in 10,000 chance of Charlie improving from nucleoside therapy and then being able to interact with his parents, perhaps with enough improvement in his breathing so that he could leave the intensive care unit. That chance is small, but the alternative for Charlie was death (Professor Hirano cited this as justification for offering experimental treatment). Some people would regard it as rational to take the risk and embark on the experimental treatment in the face of those odds.

One way of making rational choices in the face of uncertainty is to draw on decision theory. This is a mathematical approach that combines the probability of different outcomes with the value assigned to different outcomes. It assesses the expected value of different choices, and can sometimes help to work out which is the better choice. As a simple example, if you bought a lottery ticket for one pound, hoping to win £5 million pounds, this would be a rational choice only if the chance of a winning ticket were more than 1 in 5 million. Of course (and this is not likely to be a surprise), the actual chance of winning the jackpot in the lottery is typically much smaller than this, and lottery tickets, by and large, do not represent rational choices or sound investment strategies. What of the more complex situation of a patient facing death without treatment, or several months of pain and discomfort with a 1 in 10,000 chance of improvement? In that situation, assuming a 1 in 10,000 chance of survival with full quality of life (with a value of '1') for, say 70 years, it would be rational to undergo treatment for 3 months with a negative value of at most −0.03. This negative value is very small and only just less than zero. On the face of it, this seems like it would potentially rule out such a gamble where treatment would involve a significant amount of suffering.

However, there is no obvious objective way to arrive at quality of life scores for the pain and discomfort arising from medical treatment. They are derived, typically, from the preferences of people reflecting on treatment options. If some people would take the gamble and choose painful treatment, even where it has only a 1 in 10,000 chance of leading to survival with acceptable quality of life, that implies that the negative value they place on treatment is within this threshold value (of −0.03). That might mean that we need to revise our view of how bad it is to receive painful treatment.

Alternatively, we might question the soundness of their decisions. Where people's actual decisions deviate from what standard decision theory recommends, we might be tempted to question whether their behaviour is rational. Perhaps they are wrong to choose treatment? However, we know from the widespread popularity of lotteries (as well as other forms of gambling) that people do not always make choices that maximise expected utility. Some philosophers have suggested that, given that many intuitive choices do not map onto decision theory, we need a broader view about what counts as rational. Lara Buchak has argued that rational choices are a function of the probability of different outcomes; that is, the value that is placed on them, but also on how individuals trade off value between worst-case and best-case scenarios.[34] Some people are more concerned for the potential benefits of treatment (survival, improvement) than the potential downsides. Others are worried much more about the downsides than the benefits. We know that people vary in their attitudes towards risk. Some are risk averse, while others are relatively risk tolerant, or may even seek out risks, relishing the opportunity to achieve large gains (even at low probability). 'Risk-weighted expected utility maximisation', as advocated by Buchak, is a more complicated model of decision-making that accommodates a wider range of choices. Perhaps we shouldn't be surprised if some parents make choices that judges or doctors wouldn't share.

Another dominant approach was introduced by political philosopher John Rawls. As an alternative to maximising expected utility (decision theory and utilitarianism), he introduced the concept of 'maximin'.[35] According to this approach, it would be rational to make choices that would safeguard the worst-case scenario. Where outcomes are uncertain, we should make the worst outcome as least bad as possible. Applying maximin to the case of Charlie Gard, we should ask not what the chance is of the best outcome (improvement or even cure), rather how bad 3 months of intensive care would be compared with death now. Is the badness of 3 months of intensive care worse than death? If the answer is yes, then a trial of treatment should not be provided. If the answer is no, then the trial should be conducted, even if the chances are very small of it succeeding. According to maximin, whether a choice is worth choosing will turn not on the magnitude of the chance of success but on how bad the downsides of the choice are compared to the alternatives.

Maximin coheres in many ways with ordinary choice. Returning to the lottery example, maximin predicts people will choose lotteries as long as the loss is sustainable. The loss together with the hope is, for many people, better than the status quo. The actual chance of winning is largely irrelevant to people.

Another reason why decision makers might vary in their approach to treatment with a low chance of benefit arises from their different perspectives. Patients who are faced with their own death, or parents who are in the terrible position of contemplating the death of their child, are thinking about a single case, a single roll of the dice, if you like. Treatment will work, or it won't. There is a sense in which the statistics are irrelevant. After all, the child cannot be 0.0001% alive.

In contrast, doctors in intensive care, paediatric oncologists or other specialists caring for children with serious illness may be quite frequently in a position where a child is dying despite medical treatment. In that situation, if they embark on further treatment that is unlikely to help, we can expect that most of the time it won't do any good. If the treatments are unpleasant or associated with side effects, most children that the doctors treat will be harmed by that treatment, but will still die. Occasionally, a child will improve.

Take the hypothetical example given earlier of a treatment that has only a 1 in 10,000 chance of working but will cause some months of pain and discomfort. From the doctor's point of view, if they provide treatment with those odds, they can expect to see many, many patients being harmed and only very rare patients benefiting. Out of 10,000 patients, 9999 would experience the negatives of the treatment, while only one would experience any positive.

From a doctor's perspective, such a treatment is a very poor investment. Indeed, this sort of perspective is important if we are thinking about provision of healthcare resources. (We will return to that in the next chapter.) However, even if there is no resource scarcity (indeed, even if there isn't any issue about the cost of treatment), it might seem legitimate for the health professional or the judge to look at the wider rule or principle. What would be the effect of a policy or a principle that allowed treatment with low probability of benefit? If, in cases like that of Charlie Gard, doctors provide treatments that have a low probability of working and a high probability of causing harm, that will mean that they will be responsible for harming many children while benefiting only very few. That seems to provide some reason not to agree to parents' requests, even if those requests are understandable and rational. (Of course, this depends on the theory of weighing risks and harms that one accepts. On standard decision theory, doctors should not provide any treatment which has a greater than 50/50 chance of causing more harm than benefit. On maximin, it will depend on how bad the harms are and what the alternatives are.)

This argument assumes that treatment would overall be harmful and worse than death for the children who don't improve. We have already seen that in contested cases – like that of Charlie Gard – there can be considerable disagreement about whether the children are suffering, and if so, how much. If treatment wouldn't cause much discomfort, or is unlikely to cause discomfort, that may change the equation in terms of the number of children harmed and the reasonableness of a policy or general approach. One possibility might be to apply a more complicated model of outcomes. We could imagine for example, that there is a 1 in 10,000 chance of treatment leading to benefit, while there is a 1 in 100 chance of causing significant suffering. Perhaps there is a larger chance (1 in 10) that treatment would cause some (lower) suffering, and a higher chance that any suffering could be relieved by medicines? Treatment with these sorts of outcomes, applied on a large scale (10,000 children), would lead to 1 child benefiting, but 100 suffering significantly, 1000 experiencing some suffering, and 8899 experiencing neither benefit nor harm.

How much consideration should we give to this argument? For competent adult patients, there may be only a limited role for this sort of concern. If there is good reason to think that treatment could be of benefit, and the patient judges that benefit (even if unlikely) to be sufficient, then potentially the doctor should provide it – even if adopting this approach in similar cases means that many patients will be harmed.[h] (We will consider in the next chapter the separate resources-related reason against allowing this sort of treatment.) For children, though, that doesn't seem like the right approach. It is legitimate to limit some parental choices that will predictably cause harm to children. However, that still leaves open the question of how much harm, and how likely/unlikely a benefit would be reasonable. We will return to thinking about where the boundaries of reasonable parental decisions should be drawn in Chapter 6.

Hierarchy of reasons

In this chapter, we have explored some of the different factors that it is important to weigh when trying to assess whether prolonging life with medical treatment would be in a child's best interests. We have looked at situations where a child's future life is limited in quantity or in quality, where there may be the prospect of suffering from treatment, where there may be a reduced probability of improvement or survival or where treatment could be thought by some to lead to a less dignified death.

As we have analysed these different factors, it is clear that some are more clear-cut, while others are more controversial or contested.[i] For example, when thinking about a child with limited quantity of life, the argument against providing treatment is clearest where a child is imminently dying (or has already died). For a child who may survive for a period of weeks or months, there might be different reasonable views about whether that benefit is enough to outweigh the burdens of treatment. Thinking about quality of life, the argument against treatment is strongest where there is very good reason to believe that the treatment will cause the child to suffer significantly, or that they will experience severe suffering from their underlying illness. However, there may be much more disagreement about whether or not treatment would be in the child's interests in situations where the child isn't suffering but is experiencing reduced benefit from life. There may be, indeed there are likely to be, different views about what degree of awareness or cognition is enough to make treatment worth providing and life (for the child) potentially worth prolonging. Although there are good reasons for health professionals to be chary of providing treatment with very low chance of benefit (since, as a policy, this may harm many children), again, there may be different views about how low a chance would be too low. In contrast, the concern for dignity in

---

[h]Agreeing to provide the treatment does not mean recommending the treatment. The doctor may be justified in this sort of situation in advising the patient against embarking on unpleasant treatments that have low chance of benefit.

[i]In the 'taxonomy' provided by the RCPCH, the higher subcategories are more clear-cut than those that are lower down in the list.

dying or in death appeared to be one that could not provide a distinct clear argument against treatment.

We have tried to think about these different factors in isolation. In practice, though, they may occur together. That may make things easier. The most clear-cut case for life-prolonging treatment not being in a child's best interests is likely to be where that would provide little benefit (because of reduction in both quantity and quality of life) and cause suffering. Where that is the case, there may be least scope for reasonable disagreement.

Where things are not clear-cut, where there is reasonable debate about whether the scales are tipped in one direction or the other, we should generally give the benefit of the doubt and provide treatment. That reflects the general philosophy in medicine of prolonging life. It is also a decision that can be revised or revisited if more evidence accumulates. (Whereas a decision not to provide life-prolonging treatment often cannot be undone once taken.) It means, in many cases, that doctors should potentially accommodate and respect parents' views about treatment for a child, even if they do not share that view.

But just because treatment is potentially in a child's interests, that is not the end of the matter. It may not be able to be ethically provided. There is something else that we need to take into account.

References

1. Larcher, V., Craig, F., Bhogal, K., Wilkinson, D. & Brierley, J. (2015) Making decisions to limit treatment in life-limiting and life-threatening conditions in children: a framework for practice. *Arch Dis Child*, 100, s1-23. (This guideline was co-authored by DW, who provided the original draft taxonomy.)
2. Sinnott-Armstrong, W. & Miller, F. G. (2013) What makes killing wrong? *J Med Ethics*, 39, 3-7.
3. Truog, R. D. (2010) Is it always wrong to perform futile CPR? *N Engl J Med*, 362, 477-9.
4. Paris, J. J., P. Angelos, and M. D. Schreiber. (2010) Does compassion for a family justify providing futile CPR?. *J Perinatol* 30 (12):770-2.
5. *Great Ormond Street Hospital v Yates & Ors* [2017] EWHC 972 (Fam) (11 April 2017). Para 15
6. Re A (A Child) [2015] *EWHC 443 (Fam)*. Para 26
7. *Aintree University Hospital NHS Foundation Trust v. James* [2013] UKSC 67.
8. Kings College Hospital NHS Foundation Trust and MH [2015] *EWHC 1920 (Fam)*.
9. Thomas, D. & Jones, D. (1971) *The poems of Dylan Thomas*. Edited with an introduction and notes by Daniel Jones. (Second printing.) New York, New Directions Publishing Corporation.
10. Kamm, F. M. (2017) Advanced and end of life care: cautionary suggestions. *J Med Ethics* 43 (9):577-586.
11. Lawrence, J. (1998) Child B: the truth about her last days. *Independent*. Accessed from <http://www.independent.co.uk/life-style/child-b-the-truth-about-her-last-days-1159951.html>.
12. Herodotus, Aubrey De Selincourt, and John Marincola. 2003. *The histories. Further revised edition*. ed. London; New York: Penguin Books.
13. Re C (medical treatment) [1998] 1 FLR 384.
14. An NHS Trust v MB [2006] 2 F.L.R. 319.
15. Press Association (2016) Severely disabled baby should be allowed to die, judge rules. The Guardian. Accessed 27/4/2017 from <https://www.theguardian.com/uk-news/2016/jul/22/severely-disabled-baby-withdraw-life-support-high-court-judge-rules>.
16. Gregoretti, C., Ottonello, G., Chiarini Testa, M. B., Mastella, C., Rava, L., Bignamini, E., et al. (2013) Survival of patients with spinal muscular atrophy type 1. *Pediatrics*, 131, e1509-14.
17. Ryan, M. M., Kilham, H., Jacobe, S., Tobin, B. & Isaacs, D. (2007) Spinal muscular atrophy type 1: is long-term mechanical ventilation ethical? *J Paediatr Child Health*, 43, 237-42.
18. Gray, K., Isaacs, D., Kilham, H. A. & Tobin, B. (2013) Spinal muscular atrophy type I: do the benefits of ventilation compensate for its burdens? *Ibid*.49, 807-12.
19. Parfit, D. (1984) *Reasons and persons*. Oxford: Oxford University Press.
20. Griffin, James. (1986) *Well-being: its meaning, measurement and moral importance*. Oxford: Clarendon.
21. DeGrazia, D. (1995) Value theory and the best interests standard. *Bioethics* 9 (1):50-61.

22. Albrecht, G. L. & Devlieger, P. J. (1999) The disability paradox: high quality of life against all odds. *Soc Sci Med*, 48, 977-88.

23. Gipson, J., Kahane, G. & Savulescu, J. (2014) Attitudes of Lay People to Withdrawal of Treatment in Brain Damaged Patients. *Neuroethics*, 7, 1-9.

24. Fletcher, G. (2016) Objective list theories. in G. Fletcher (Ed.) *The Routledge handbook of philosophy of wellbeing*. Abingdon, Routledge, pp. 148-160.

25. Parfit, D. (1984) *Reasons and persons*. Oxford: Oxford University Press.

26. Wilkinson, D. (2006) Is it in the best interests of an intellectually disabled infant to die? *J Med Ethics*, 32, 454-459.

27. *A Local Health Board v Y (A Child) and Others* [2016] EWHC 206 (Fam).

28. Schmidt, M., Banzett, R. B., Raux, M., Morelot-Panzini, C., Dangers, L., Similowski, T., et al. (2014) Unrecognized suffering in the ICU: addressing dyspnea in mechanically ventilated patients. *Intensive Care Med*, 40, 1-10.

29. Alasad, J. A., Abu Tabar, N. & Ahmad, M. M. (2015) Patients' experience of being in intensive care units. *J Crit Care*, 30, 859.e7-11.

30. Rotondi, A. J., Chelluri, L., Sirio, C., Mendelsohn, A., Schulz, R., Belle, S., et al. (2002) Patients' recollections of stressful experiences while receiving prolonged mechanical ventilation in an intensive care unit. *Crit Care Med*, 30, 746-52.

31. Fink, R. M., Makic, M. B., Poteet, A. W. & Oman, K. S. (2015) The Ventilated Patient's Experience. *Dimens Crit Care Nurs*, 34, 301-8.

32. Kozlowski, L. J., Kost-Byerly, S., Colantuoni, E., Thompson, C. B., Vasquenza, K. J., Rothman, S. K., et al. (2014) Pain prevalence, intensity, assessment and management in a hospitalized pediatric population. *Pain Manag Nurs*, 15, 22-35.

33. Great Ormond Street Hospital for Children. (2017, 13/7/17). '*GOSH's position statement, hearing on 13 July 2017.*' From <http://www.gosh.nhs.uk/file/23611/download?token=aTPZchww>.

34. Buchak, L. (2017) Why high-risk, non-expected-utility-maximising gambles can be rational and beneficial: the case of HIV cure studies. *J Med Ethics*, 43, 90-95.

35. Rawls, John. (1999) *A theory of justice*. Rev. ed. Oxford: Oxford University Press.

CHAPTER 4

Resources

> *'There was an old man of Kilkenny*
> *Who never had more than a penny*
> *He spent all that money, in onions and honey*
> *That wayward old man of Kilkenny.'*
> **Edward Lear**

> *'Taking Three as the subject to reason about—*
> *A convenient number to state—*
> *We add Seven, and Ten, and then multiply out*
> *By One Thousand diminished by Eight.*
> *The result we proceed to divide, as you see,*
> *By Nine Hundred and Ninety and Two:*
> *Then subtract Seventeen, and the answer must be*
> *Exactly and perfectly true.'*
> **The Hunting of the Snark, Lewis Carroll**

'It is imperative that I make clear that this case is not about money and, if anyone were to suggest that Charlie would have nucleoside treatment but for the cost, they would be completely wrong.'
JUSTICE FRANCIS, APRIL 11[1]

'The heartbreaking story of the 11-month-old Charlie Gard in England is a story of single-payer [healthcare] … a government program that says, "No, we're going to remove life support from your precious 11-month-old child because the government has decided that the prospects of their life are such that they no longer warrant an investment in health services."'
US VICE PRESIDENT MIKE PENCE, JULY 10[2]

We noted at the end of the previous chapter that, even if treatment is possibly in the interests of a child, there may be another reason not to provide it – the problem of limited healthcare resources. Was Charlie Gard denied treatment because of distributive justice, because of rationing of publicly funded healthcare? As the quotes above make clear, there were opposing views about that in the Gard case. Examining that question will help us understand the wider relevance of resources in disputes about treatment.

We will start by outlining why resources are relevant to decisions about providing treatment like intensive care. Intensive care is a scarce and expensive medical resource. We will then return to the Gard case and argue that, despite the claims of the judge and some commentators, the Gard case was at least partly about resources. The cost (or scarcity) of treatment cannot be ignored, either for this case or for other cases. The very substantial challenge is that, at present, there is no clear process for taking into account limited resources in decisions about provision of intensive care. In the second half of the chapter, we will consider how or when cost limitations would justify not providing life-prolonging treatment like intensive care. We will explain how cost-effectiveness might be used to derive some practical heuristics for when intensive care should or should not be provided. Finally, we will argue that there is a need to balance competing values (and competing conceptions of wellbeing and quality of life) in allocation of intensive care beds and other limited healthcare resources.

PART ONE

Why are resources relevant to decisions about intensive care?

The word 'resource' comes originally from old French – referring to a spring or source of water (literally 'rising up'). We still use the word in that way to refer to natural resources (for example, water or minerals). The word is also often used to refer to a source of value or wealth, or sometimes to valuable skills (as in 'resourceful').

'Intensive care' is a type of medical support applied to very sick patients – often replacing the function of one or more vital organs (e.g., lungs, heart, kidney). It is a medical specialty involving a set of specialised skills. It is also a physical place in the hospital where certain types of medical technology and organ support are available.

There are two features of intensive care that are relevant to it as a resource. The first is that providing intensive care is very expensive. It typically costs somewhere between £1000 and £2000 per day to provide this sort of treatment. The second, is that intensive care is scarce: in most parts of the world, there are limits to the availability of intensive care. There are only a fixed number of intensive care beds in a hospital, a set amount of specialised equipment and a finite number of staff available to provide the treatment. In many places, the demand for intensive care outstrips supply – meaning that not all patients referred for intensive care are able to be accepted.[3]

The cost and scarcity of intensive care are obviously related. If intensive care were less expensive, it would be possible for hospitals to purchase more beds and equipment or employ more staff.

These features of intensive care are ethically relevant because they mean that treatment of one patient can potentially harm one or more other patients by denying them lifesaving treatment. That is easy to see in a public healthcare system because there is a set amount of money to spend on providing healthcare for a population. Once that budget is reached, hospitals have to cancel some services, forego needed improvements or decline to provide other treatments, in an attempt to balance the books. It is no different from the situation that everyone faces when managing their own finances. If you spend very large sums on one thing (a large mortgage, a new car or an expensive holiday), other things can't be afforded. Something has to give. Spending money on highly expensive treatment for some can mean that other medical treatments cannot be provided.

As a simple analogy, imagine a chocolate cake that is shared out between a group of hungry people. We would potentially want to divide up the cake fairly so that there are equal shares of the cake for everyone. But if one person takes an extra-large slice, or more than one slice, there will be less for everyone else.

The worry is that providing highly expensive intensive care treatment to some patients may mean that other patients are denied their slice of the cake – they are not able to receive treatment. For example, artificial ventilation is extremely expensive to provide over a long period. It is estimated to cost around £600,000 to provide a year of treatment on a ventilator in intensive care.[4] It is slightly cheaper for children to receive that treatment at home, but still costs £240,000 per year. This figure is almost ten times higher than the usual maximum cost of affordable treatment in the National Health Service (NHS).[a]

Besides the actual cost of treatment, intensive care is a scarce resource. There are only a limited number of specialist paediatric intensive care beds, and a limited number of specialist medical and nursing staff available to care for children. In intensive care units (ICUs) like Great Ormond Street Hospital, it is not uncommon for doctors to have to cancel major elective surgery (for example heart surgery) because the ICU is full, and it would not be possible to provide medical care for the child after the operation. Children in ICUs in other parts of the country may not be able to be transferred to Great Ormond Street for specialist treatment or opinions. For example, in November 2016 (when Charlie was being considered by the ethics committee for long-term ventilation), 88% of paediatric intensive care beds and 84% of adult intensive care beds in England were occupied.[5] The UK recommends that ICUs should normally operate at 70% of their maximum capacity so that they are able to accommodate surges in demand.[6] In that month, 404 urgent operations in England were cancelled because of lack of capacity in adult and paediatric critical care units (16 operations were cancelled more than once). Great Ormond Street ICU itself reported in that month that 95% of its paediatric intensive care beds were occupied.[7]

Limited availability of treatment is a bigger problem for treatment in hospital in intensive care than it is for home ventilation. Nevertheless, the two are related. Children who are on home ventilation need highly specialised nursing care. Often, that is provided by former ICU nurses (who are then no longer available to help in the ICU). It is also often difficult to find, train and retain the specialist staff needed to care for a child on a ventilator at home. In that situation, the child might remain in hospital in the ICU for a long time while waiting to be able to go home. (In the case of Yasmin, discussed in the previous chapter, inability to provide treatment at home meant that she remained a patient in hospital for more than 8 years, utilising a scarce resource that no doubt affected the care of other children.)

What about treatment outside a public healthcare system? It is perhaps harder to see why resources might be relevant to decisions about treatment in a private healthcare system. After all, if a patient is paying for the treatment, they won't be taking any money out of the finite public healthcare budget. Whether intensive care costs £10 a day or £10,000 a day, this would not subtract from money available to treat other patients.

This does, however, depend on the nature of the funding. If treatment is funded through health insurance, the costs are spread amongst those who are insured. Providing highly expensive treatment for one patient or a subgroup of patients means either that the insurer is not able to meet other expenses or that future premiums will have to rise. If they were aware of the facts and the costs, it has been suggested that few people would consent to their health insurance providing treatment at very high cost for very low benefit to others (sometimes referred to as 'non–cost-worthy care').[8] On that basis, prudent insurance schemes would be justified in imposing some limits on treatment and in assuming that those who take up insurance consent to those limits. (If you have ever attempted to read the fine print of your own car, home or health insurance policy, you will be acutely aware that all insurance schemes set limits on what they will and will not cover.)

---

[a]This is set at approximately £30,000 per quality-adjusted life year. We will return later to some of the ethical challenges in assessing quality of life. However, of note, the cost of long-term mechanical ventilation substantially exceeds the cost limit for treatment, even if we totally ignore any question of quality of life.

Moreover, even if a patient is funding treatment completely from their own pocket, the aforementioned scarcity of intensive care means that there could still be good reason to limit intensive care that is of low benefit. Even in private hospitals, there are times when the ICU is full. This may be more likely in highly specialised centres that treat patients with complex or rare conditions from a wide geographic area. One US paediatric intensive care consultant (in a large, tertiary intensive care) described to us the problem that he faces:

> '*Every morning in the ICU we count our anticipated discharges and our scheduled post-ops (children scheduled for semi-elective procedures who will need ICU care post-operatively). We admit emergency cases and scheduled post-ops until we are full, then we cancel the remaining surgeries and divert emergencies to other hospitals ... We have 30 beds and are always full.*'[9]

Next, the time and attention of specialist doctors and nurses devoted to one patient may mean that there is less time and attention for other patients. Finally, there is a complex interplay between public and private investment in healthcare. Robert Truog, reflecting on the Gard case, noted that '[t]he very existence of tertiary care medical centers that are able to do the research and provide the care requested by Charlie's parents depends on the vast communal investment that has been made by society in the infrastructure of our health care system over many decades.'[10] Because of the past public investment in developing healthcare and in performing research, all within a community have a stake in how healthcare is provided. Looking forward, if we accept or allow our health systems to provide treatment of very low benefit, the total cost (both privately and publicly funded) of the systems will rise substantially. Total healthcare expenditure in the US is projected to reach $5.5 trillion by 2025, almost 20% of Gross Domestic Product.[11] If societies wish to rein in some of these ever-escalating costs, they must accept some limits to the treatment that is provided – even in private healthcare.

Resources and treatment disputes

Twenty-two years before the case of Charlie Gard, there was intense media attention on another case of disagreement about medical treatment for a seriously ill child in the UK. The main debate in that case focused specifically on the question of finite healthcare resources.

In 1995, David Bowen sought an experimental treatment for his 10-year-old daughter Jaymee. At age 6, Jaymee had received treatment for lymphoma. However, 3 years later she had developed a second cancer – acute myeloid leukaemia. Despite chemotherapy and a bone marrow transplant, Jaymee had developed a relapse in early 1995, and doctors advised her family that she had only 6 to 8 weeks to live.[12]

Faced with this news, David Bowen, in a similar way to Connie Yates and Chris Gard, had conducted his own research and contacted specialists overseas. Two US specialists based in California recommended a second bone marrow transplant for Jaymee, while an adult cancer specialist at Hammersmith hospital in London indicated that he would support treatment with chemotherapy, followed by a transplant if the chemotherapy was successful.[13] The London specialist estimated that chemotherapy would have a 10% to 20% chance of achieving remission (allowing a transplant). The estimated cost of the treatment was £75,000.

The local health authority (Cambridge) had a responsibility for contracting health services outside its geographic area. The Director of Public Health from the authority, Dr Zimmern, wrote to Jaymee's father in February 1995. At that time, the stated concern about treatment was based on an assessment of Jaymee's best interests:

> '*I should like to emphasise that any decision on this issue will be taken in the light of all the clinical advice available to it in the context of [Department of Health] guidance on the funding of*

unproven or experimental treatments, at all times with [Jaymee's] best interest in mind ...
Should there be any misunderstanding I should state quite clearly that any decision ... will be
made taking all clinical and other matters into consideration and not on financial grounds.'[13]

Shortly after that letter, the Authority officially declined to approve the treatment. Her father
objected to the Authority's decision. He believed that a small chance of success was a calculated
gamble worth taking.[14] David Bowen sought a judicial review of the basis of the Authority's
decision. In an affidavit to the High Court, Dr Zimmern provided a different justification for its
decision:

'Having considered all the medical opinions put before me I decided to accept the clinical judgment
of Drs Broadbent, Pinkerton and Mellor that a further course of intensive chemotherapy with a
view to a second transplant operation was not in the best interests of [Jaymee]. I have also been
influenced in my decision by the consistent advice and directions of the Department of Health with
regard to the funding of treatments which have not been proven to be of benefit.... The doctors to
whom I spoke were consistent in their advice that the proposed treatment was neither standard
nor had been formally evaluated. I also considered that the substantial expenditure on treatment
with such small prospect of success would not be an effective use of resources. The amount of funds
available for health care are not limitless. The [authority] has a responsibility to ensure that
sufficient funds are available from their limited resources for the provision of treatment for other
patients which is likely to be effective.'[13]

When the case was first heard in the High Court, the judge (Laws) said that Jaymee's fundamental
right to life required that the Health Authority show compelling objective reasons for giving other
patients priority over her. He said that it was not sufficient to state merely that resources were
limited. He asked the health authority to reconsider its decision, noting that he found it hard to
imagine a proper basis for withholding the treatment.

However, this decision was not upheld in the Court of Appeal.

Sir Thomas Bingham acknowledged that 'difficult and agonizing judgments have to be made
as to how a limited budget is best allocated to the maximum advantage of the maximum number
of patients'.[13] The judges felt that the Authority had weighed the evidence given to it about
treatment, and that there was no basis for overruling its decision.

In the High Court and in the Court of Appeal, arguments about treatment for Jaymee
Bowen centred on the question of allocation of limited resources, not on her best interests, and
whether the health authority was justified in declining to fund treatment. While the judges were
sympathetic to David and Jaymee Bowen's plight, they expressed their reluctance to substitute
their own decision for that of the health authority. The question of how to allocate resources was
'not a judgment which the court can make'.[13]

This reflects a wider principle that limits the involvement of courts in resource allocation in the
UK. Barrister and legal academic Charles Foster, analysing the UK legal approach to healthcare
resource allocation, has put it starkly: 'The law is very simple. The courts will not interfere with
a decision about how money is allocated unless that decision is frankly irrational'.[15]

Two reasons

In the Bowen case, the court and media focus was on the question of limited resources. However,
in interviews about the case after it had concluded, a number of the medical specialists involved
expressed anger and dismay that this was a distortion of the debate. Their central concern had
always been about what would be in Jaymee's best interests.[16] They felt that further chemotherapy and a repeat bone marrow transplant would be wrong, and would do more harm than

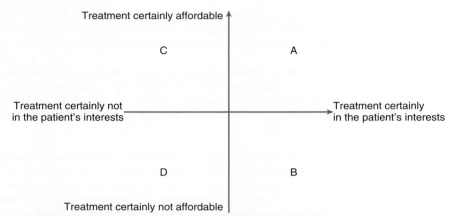

Fig. 4.1 Affordability and best interests: two reasons against treatment.

good. As we saw in the previous chapter, at the age of 11, having received the transplant from private funding, Jaymee appeared to disagree with that view and was grateful for having received her treatment.

In the conclusion to Chapter 2, we mentioned two core ethical justifications for doctors refusing to provide a medical treatment. The first is that treatment would harm the patient, while the second is that providing treatment would harm other patients (particularly by preventing them from being able to access beneficial medical treatment). These two ethical reasons might coincide, or they might come apart. Fig. 4.1 shows the relationship between the two.

If treatment were both affordable and in a child's interests (region A in the Fig. 4.1), doctors should definitely provide it. If treatment were neither affordable nor in the child's interests (region D), treatment should not be started or should be stopped. We could call this a 'doubly harmful' situation (treatment would harm the child and other children). Sometimes the picture is more mixed. Imagine a highly expensive drug for a severe illness that has no side effects but only a very slim chance of helping the patient. In that case, it seems clear that there would be little for the patient to lose by receiving the treatment. It would not harm them to be given the treatment. But it may be completely unaffordable for a publicly funded health system. The treatment would be in region B in the figure. Alternatively, we could imagine a situation where a treatment would be very cheap (perhaps because the parents are proposing to pay for it themselves) but would definitely harm a child (region C).

Most cases of disputed treatment that come before the courts in the UK potentially fall into the 'doubly harmful' category. That is because they are often about providing a scarce and expensive treatment (intensive care), and they are situations where the treatment is likely not to help the patient, or to do more harm than good.

In the affidavit to the court, Dr Zimmern wrote that he had accepted the clinical judgment of several specialists that the requested treatment was not in Jaymee's best interests. However, he had 'also been influenced' by concern about limited resources. This appears to acknowledge the double harm of treatment. Yet, the legal argument in the Bowen case focused only on the second of these justifications – on the resource question.

This is the opposite to most other cases of disputed treatment in the UK. In those cases, courts have focused exclusively on the best interests question and ignored or set aside any consideration of resources. As Justice Francis in the case of Charlie Gard was at pains to note, this reflects the jurisdiction of the court in a situation of a disagreement about what would be best for a child. It is clear from previous cases and from the Children Act that 'the welfare of the child is paramount'.[17] Justice Francis stated forcefully that 'this case is not about money'.[1]

Does it matter which argument or reason is the basis for not providing treatment? It could be very important for the implications of decisions. If treatment is certainly not in a child's best interests, then doctors shouldn't provide it, even if parents can afford to pay for it. On the other hand, if the main reason not to provide treatment is because of the cost, then it may be ethical to provide the treatment if the problem of affordability can be resolved.

In Jaymee Bowen's case, support from a private donor meant that she was able to receive privately funded treatment from the specialist in London. (In the event, she received a different experimental treatment – donor lymphocyte infusion, rather than a repeat bone marrow transplantation – and died from graft versus host disease in March 1997.)[18]

But what if the two arguments (harm to the patient and harm to others) point in the same direction? We might think that it doesn't matter if the courts focus only on one of them because they both mean the same thing.

One concern is that the exclusion of questions of resources means that doctors and courts have to concentrate on an argument that is much more difficult to make. As we saw in Chapter 3, it is very challenging to know how to weigh up the possible benefits of nucleoside treatment against the uncertain harms of intensive care. We highlighted just how challenging it is to assess when life might not be worth living, or when a state of disability is sufficiently severe that it is not in a child's interests to remain alive.

By contrast, the question of distributive justice and harm to others is much clearer. To see why that might be case, we could consider an analogy. Imagine that you are looking at an individual and considering whether or not they are tall. To answer that question, you would need to have some definition in your mind about what counts as tall. There would potentially be different views about that definition, but it would also depend in part on the context (e.g., are they male or female, are they an adult or child, what country or community do they come from?). There may be clear cases, but there are also likely to be borderline cases where it is not clear whether the person should be considered tall or not. Any cutoff point that we used to decide would be, at least to some degree, arbitrary. Now imagine that there are two people that you are looking at, and you are asked 'who is taller?' Compared with the first question, this isn't difficult in the slightest. There might still be cases where it is hard to say (where they are very similar in height). But most of the time we wouldn't expect there to be much debate or disagreement. We do not need to agree on some arbitrary definition to decide which person is taller.

In a similar way, it may be unclear whether spending a large sum of money on experimental treatment or continuing intensive care would benefit a single patient. But there are many situations where that same amount of money or the same intensive care bed could help another patient more. One potential explanation for why the Jaymee Bowen legal case centred on resources is because the legal team reached a view that this argument was more likely to be successful.[19] Indeed, it was successful in the courtroom. Notwithstanding the strong views of some of the medical specialists caring for Jaymee, it was simply unclear whether or not further treatment was in her best interests. Yet, on the basis of the high cost of treatment and low chance of benefit, the health authority was clearly justified in declining to provide public funding for it. That was certainly the view of the Court of Appeal.

Were resources relevant to Charlie Gard?

But what about the Gard case?

There were two separate resources associated with the treatment requested by Charlie's parents. The first was the nucleoside replacement therapy, while the second related to the provision of intensive care necessary to keep Charlie alive during a trial of experimental therapy. Nucleoside replacement therapy itself was relatively inexpensive (one quote put the cost at several hundred pounds a month) and not in short supply. The intensive care element of treatment, though, as already noted, was both expensive and scarce.

On the surface, it appears that resources did not play a role for decisions about Charlie Gard. There are several reasons in support of this view. The first and most obvious is that Charlie's parents had raised funds to take him out of the public healthcare system to receive treatment overseas. So, there would have been no basis for refusing that request as a form of rationing within the UK health system. In fact, concern for limited resources actually provided a reason to allow Charlie's parents to take him overseas. The fundraising campaign for Charlie's treatment reached its goal on the 2nd of April, the day before his High Court hearing was due to begin.[20] Yet, Charlie continued to receive treatment in intensive care within the NHS for almost another 4 months. If he had been transferred to the US in April, the intensive care bed that he was occupying could have been available for other children much earlier. It is not clear what the costs of Charlie's medical treatment were at Great Ormond Street. However, based on an estimated cost of £1300 per day in intensive care, continued treatment seems likely to have cost more than £150,000. In addition, the legal costs of taking Charlie's case to the court (and then of the subsequent appeals) are not publicly available, but they were also likely to have been considerable. (In one NHS case that went to the High Court and Court of Appeal, the legal costs were approximately £50,000.)[21]

Of course, it is always easy in retrospect. At the time that doctors at Great Ormond Street prepared to go to court, it might have been expected that Charlie's case would go through one court hearing and not three levels of appeal (plus an additional high court hearing). The doctors and the hospital no doubt hoped that it would be possible to reach an agreement or a decision much sooner than actually happened. So some of the costs of the legal dispute (and of prolonged provision of treatment) might not have been able to be anticipated.

However, as a general principle, the case highlights that it can sometimes be a better use of the finite resources of a public healthcare system to provide a treatment for a fixed period of time (rather than engaging in a costly legal dispute) or to allow a request to access the treatment (overseas or privately funded), even if the medical judgment is that the treatment would have little or no benefit.

The second reason that resources did not appear to be an issue in the Gard case is that, at the start of January, the British doctors were preparing to provide the requested treatment to Charlie. They had made an application to their clinical ethics committee and had a plan for him to have a tracheostomy. They were apparently going to pay for treatment within the NHS. The reason that did not go ahead was not because of a resource shortfall, nor because the ICU was full. It was because the doctors treating Charlie had come to believe that there was no chance of the treatment working.

The third reason is, as noted earlier, that the court was not asked to make a decision about the provision of healthcare resources for Charlie. As we noted previously, the entire focus of the High Court decision in April was on the basis of what was perceived to be best for Charlie. The only mention of the costs of treatment was to reject its significance for the decision.

However, even if resources were not directly implicated in the decision about Charlie, they might have played a role indirectly. Indeed, a decision to deny Charlie Gard access to experimental treatment in the UK would arguably have been more solidly and defensibly made on grounds of limitation of resources and distributive justice.

Resource implications of single case versus multiple cases

GENERAL PRINCIPLES AND CONSISTENCY

When disputes about treatment arise, there is usually a great deal of attention paid to the specific circumstances of the case. In court cases, the judges will sometimes emphasise that they are not deriving general principles but are considering the particular child and what would be in this child's best interests. If we apply a similar single-patient approach to the question of resource use, that may sometimes seem to undermine the case against providing treatment. It might be, for example, that at a particular point in time there isn't a high demand on beds in intensive care. In paediatric and adult ICUs, there is a high seasonal peak of activity relating to viral illness over winter. If a child needed intensive care over the summer, there might be sufficient beds available that surgery wouldn't need to be cancelled or admissions refused.

Next, if we are thinking about expense, while the costs of treatment may accumulate over time, the total cost of care may represent only a small fraction of the healthcare budget of an individual hospital or healthcare system. As an example, according to Great Ormond Street's annual report, the total operating expenses of the hospital in 2016 were of the order of £400 million.[22] The estimated cost of 3 months of intensive care for Charlie Gard would represent less than 0.03% of the total hospital budget.

Alternatively, it may be difficult to prove that treatment of one patient will lead to another patient being denied treatment. In the Jaymee Bowen case, the judge in the High Court criticised the health authority for failing to make a clear case that other patients would be harmed by providing Jaymee's requested treatment. It is part of the diffuse nature of large budgets that spending in one area doesn't necessarily lead to a direct (and equal) reduction in another. It may be spread out over many areas (or many patients) so that the individual impact is small. According to the public records, Great Ormond Street Hospital did not have to cancel any urgent elective surgery in November 2016 (nor in the following months while Charlie was in intensive care).[b]

However, when we consider questions of resources, we have a responsibility to look beyond the individual case. It is the same principle that applies when we think about other limited resources. For example, when there is a drought and water reservoir levels are very low, people in the community are sometimes asked to conserve water – for example, by avoiding watering their garden, or by washing the car from a bucket rather than using a hose. In this sort of situation, we might be tempted to focus on only one particular instance. For example, I could look at my wilting flowers or browning lawn and think that there would be no harm done if I water them. I might try to rationalise that surely it couldn't have any appreciable impact on the water levels in the reservoir? But if everyone had the same attitude, the reservoir levels would certainly fall, and the problem of scarce water for the community would worsen. Since we are dealing with a shared community resource (intensive care beds, equipment, staff), it is important to apply the same principles in every case. In the Bowen case, the judge in the Court of Appeal made the

---

[b]There are no records indicating whether less urgent surgery was cancelled or delayed over this period. There are also no publicly available records of how often patients might have been declined admission to the intensive care unit because of lack of capacity.[23]

point that in individual cases it was neither necessary nor possible to demonstrate the direct impact of allocation on other patients:

> *'it would be totally unrealistic to require the Authority to come to the court with its accounts and seek to demonstrate that if this treatment were provided for B then there would be a patient, C, who would have to go without treatment. No major Authority could run its financial affairs in a way which would permit such a demonstration.'*[13]

There are two reasons, then, why we have a responsibility to consider the wider application of principles or the wider implications of a single case. First, the impact on our scarce resource will be magnified if it is applied in more than one case. The amount of water used in garden watering is small if I do it, but large if everyone does it. The impact on intensive care beds may be small for an individual case, but very large if ICUs regularly provide treatment with very low benefit.

We also need to consider fairness. It would be unfair of me to break the rules and water my garden, but to expect everyone else to apply the rules strictly. Similarly, even if we think in a particular case that we might be generous and provide the expensive/scarce treatment to a child – to Charlie Gard, for example – it would be unfair not to apply the same approach in other cases. What about other children with rare conditions and low chances of improvement? Surely they are equally deserving of treatment?

One important reason, then, for doctors and hospitals to oppose treatment in Charlie's case was because of the general principle that there is a need to impose limits on expensive treatment of low benefit in other similar cases. Although the attention was on Charlie, and the arguments were about Charlie's specific circumstances, the justification could have been at least in part based on the implications for other children. In fact, as public attention to the case became more intense, this concern arguably became even more relevant (though it could not be publicly expressed). For example, if Charlie's parents had won their appeal in the European Court and had been allowed to pursue further treatment for Charlie, it seems highly likely that this would have led to an increase in other families requesting continued intensive care or experimental treatment, and in opposing health professionals who were recommending that treatment should be stopped or withheld. It would have encouraged other families to seek media and social media support and to mount legal appeals. At the same time, this would have potentially made doctors or hospitals more reluctant to impose limits on treatment because they feared that they would ultimately be required to provide or allow treatment despite their misgivings.

The point here is that resource allocation has to take into account general principles and how they might be responsibly applied in other cases. That may have influenced decision makers who were considering whether or not to oppose treatment in Charlie's case. That doesn't necessarily make it right. For the reasons already noted, one of the distinctive features of Charlie's case (that his parents were proposing self-funded treatment outside the public healthcare system) potentially meant that general principles applying to other patients should not have been directly applied to Charlie.

PAST CASES, PRECEDENTS AND THE ZONE OF PARENTAL DISCRETION

Awareness of resource limits might have influenced doctors in Charlie's case to make a decision that could be consistently applied in other cases. Resource limits might have been relevant in another slightly different way, by influencing where courts and doctors draw the line for overruling parents.

In Chapter 6 we will discuss in more detail the idea of a 'zone' of parental discretion. This zone represents the amount of leeway that parents are given to make decisions. The boundaries of that zone are not set in stone. Clinicians, courts and the community come to understand where that boundary lies by looking at past cases of disputes and seeing when parents have been allowed to make decisions and when they have not.

One striking feature of the Gard case was the apparent difference between countries in how much discretion parents would be given over treatment. Some countries seem to defer to parents' judgments in most cases. Commentators from those countries saw the court decisions in the Gard case as examples of judicial overreach. Other countries, like the UK, seem to give much greater weight to the views of professionals. Commentators in those countries saw the Gard decision as appropriately protecting the interests of children. We will return to this in later chapters, but there are different explanations for why some countries might have a wider or narrower zone of parental discretion. One reason to give parents greater say in medical decisions would be if a society gave greater weight to parents' autonomy, or a had a more pluralistic view about what would be best for a child.

Another reason, though, is the impact of healthcare resources. Where resources are limited, health systems cannot afford to give parents substantial discretion about medical treatment. For example, countries with very limited public healthcare systems do not have vexed public debates about providing long-term home ventilation for children with severe neuromuscular disorders. That is simply not an option. Countries with more well-resourced healthcare systems may be able to afford such treatments. They can afford debate and disagreement.

This provides at least a partial explanation for why the UK has a such a clear path to the courts in cases of disputed medical treatment and why, in the majority of cases, courts have sided with health professionals and authorised withholding or withdrawal of medical treatment. A single-payer healthcare system with finite resources has to have a robust process for setting limits on treatment.

PART TWO
How should resource limits be applied to intensive care?

> 'where the question is whether the life of a … child might be saved by however slim a chance, the responsible Authority … must do more than toll the bell of tight resources …They must explain the priorities that have led them to decline to fund the treatment.' Justice Laws[13]

We have argued that resources are relevant to provision of intensive care – even in private healthcare systems. Despite initial appearances, we have pointed out that resources were relevant to a proper ethical analysis of the Charlie Gard case.

But how should decisions be made about which patient should receive life-prolonging treatment? As was powerfully argued by the first judge in the Bowen case, it is not enough for decision makers to simply cite general principles (even if these are well-founded). If life-saving treatment is to be withheld from a gravely ill patient, there needs to be a clear, relevant basis for doing so.

Triage

One setting in which it may be impossible to help all of the patients who could benefit from treatment is in an acute disaster setting with multiple casualties (for example, an earthquake or a terrorist attack). The urgency of such situations, as well as the impossibility of aiding all equally, makes it inevitable that health professionals have to choose between patients.

Emergency 'triage' is the name given to a widely accepted medical approach to situations like this – it compares simultaneous patients and directs emergency attention to those patients who have the highest chance of dying or suffering serious harm without urgent treatment, but who have some hope of being saved.[24] Some patients receive a lower triage category – those who are well enough that they can wait or so severely unwell that they will not benefit.

We could imagine a triage model being applied to intensive care referrals. Imagine, for example, that a paediatric ICU has received two referrals for life support treatment and has a single available ICU bed. There are two critically ill infants who will almost certainly die if they do not receive urgent treatment. (We will imagine for this example that there are no other ICUs able to retrieve and provide treatment for the patients.)

Infant A has a genetic disorder causing severe lung disease. The chance of survival with treatment is less than 3%.

Infant B has severe lung problems due to a temporary disorder arising at birth. The chance of survival with intensive care is potentially as high as 94%.

In a case like this, it is immediately clear to most people that the doctor should choose to admit the second infant with the higher chance of surviving. Of course, it is regrettable that she has to make this choice. It would be better if there were some way to treat both patients, but in this example, that isn't an option. When we previously conducted a survey of the general public and gave them a scenario very similar to the triage case described, almost all elected to treat the patient with the higher chance of survival. Very few elected to toss a coin to decide.[25]

A triage case is a little bit like the analogy we gave earlier of deciding which of two people are taller. We argued that this was an easier judgment than deciding whether a single person was tall.

Of course, most of the time in intensive care, clinicians do not face a stark choice between simultaneous patients. They usually make a decision about one patient at a time. This means that a triage approach to allocation of treatment is more challenging to apply. If the ICU has a bed available and receives a single referral (for infant A), the triage approach would imply that treatment should be given. But that might mean that there are no machines/staff/beds available when infant B (with better chances) is referred for treatment tomorrow.[26] Yet, if the ICU decides not to provide treatment to patient A (because they are concerned about future patients who might need treatment), they risk foregoing treatment unnecessarily. Sometimes there will be no competing patient in need of intensive care in the short term, and infant A could have been treated.

Threshold

When patients present for treatment at different points in time, doctors cannot compare them directly. Instead they need to assess, for each individual patient, whether treatment would cross a threshold level of benefit that would make treatment worth providing. Is a 3% chance of survival too low to provide intensive care? Is 10% high enough?

In Chapter 3, we considered treatment with a low chance of benefit. Thinking only about what would be best for the patient, it is extremely challenging to define what chance of improvement would mean that treatment is not in a patient's best interests. There is no obvious 'probability threshold' that would make treatment worth providing/not worth providing. If we are considering, though, a health system with limited resources, perhaps there could be a way of determining a cutoff for providing treatment? This cutoff will depend on just how expensive treatment would be. For example, it would be reasonable to provide a desired simple treatment that could save a patient's life, even if it is very unlikely to do so (for example, if there is only a 0.001% chance of this occurring), if the treatment is innocuous and cheap. On the other hand, it may be unethical to provide an extremely expensive, high-risk and burdensome treatment that has a 15% chance of saving the patient's life. The cutoff will also depend on the availability of resources within the health system. A better resourced healthcare system with many more intensive care beds and staff would be in a position to provide treatment despite a lower chance of survival.

One way that health systems attempt to objectively and consistently decide which treatments to provide is to use cost-effectiveness analysis. In a cost-effectiveness analysis, the costs of an intervention are divided by its benefits, setting up a cost-effectiveness ratio. Interventions with a lower cost-effectiveness ratio are preferred. Cost-effectiveness analysis takes into consideration two factors that are important to decision makers. The cost of treatment has direct implications for the number of individuals who are able to benefit from health systems with a fixed budget. When alternative treatments are equally effective, choosing a less expensive treatment simply means that more patients are able to be treated. Where we are contemplating life-saving treatment, cheaper treatment means that more lives will be saved. For example, imagine that a health system has a budget of £1 million. Individuals with fatal disease A need £100,000 per treatment to cure them, while individuals with fatal disease B only need £10,000 per treatment. From that budget, policy makers would be faced with a choice of treating 10 people with disease A or 100 people with disease B. If both patient groups are similar, with similar prognoses, we should save more lives; that is, treat those with disease B.

Cost-effectiveness also takes into account the amount of health-associated value that the health system is able to promote or improve. Imagine that two treatments cost £10,000, but one will save a life, while the other will relieve a headache. It isn't controversial to think that if you have only a limited amount of money to spend, it would be better to save lives than to relieve headaches.

Cost-effectiveness analysis provides a tool for comparing treatments. But how cost-effective is cost-effective enough? Some countries and policy makers have applied a limit or threshold on cost-effectiveness to efficiently and consistently decide between different priorities. These limits are not a blanket rule. Policy makers may consider funding treatments within a range of cost-effectiveness and will often consider other factors. The idea, however, is to have a benchmark that ensures some level of consistency. In the UK, for example, interventions that cost less than a threshold level of £20,000 to £30,000 per quality-adjusted life year (QALY) are usually funded by the NHS, while those that cost more than £30,000 are not usually provided.[27]

While cost-effectiveness is not routinely used in the US for healthcare funding decisions, treatments costing more than $100,000 to $150,000 are often regarded as not offering reasonable value.[c] Cost-effectiveness has been used to inform some policy decisions around provision of treatment in the US, for example in Oregon.[30] It has also been used to justify recommendations in national evidence-based clinical guidelines and by some managed care funds.[31]

There is considerable ethical debate about the use of cost-effectiveness thresholds for deciding between different treatments, and particularly about one feature of them that attempts to place a numerical value on quality of life (so-called QALYs).[32-36] It is not our aim here to review those arguments, nor to defend cost-effectiveness analysis. Rather, the point is that cost-effectiveness thresholds are already widely used in many health systems to decide between different treatments (for example, whether new drugs will be funded). If that approach is justified, on the grounds of consistency, it may be possible to apply the same principles to deciding about intensive care.

How would this work in practice? As noted, the principle expense in the Gard case was that of providing intensive care (for a minimum of 3 months while nucleoside therapy was

---

[c]The traditional value for the cost-effectiveness threshold in the US has often been quoted as being $50,000 per QALY, though the scientific origin of this figure has been disputed.[28,29]

being trialled), costing an estimated £150,000. The best outcome estimate by the US specialist, Professor Hirano, was quoted as being a 10% chance of some improvement, albeit Charlie would still have a shortened life of severe disability.[37] If we ignore any question of quality of life (i.e., we assumed that the value of survival was full) and ignored any future costs (after 3 months), the expected value of treatment might be estimated at 10% (chance of survival) multiplied by 10 QALYs (10 years at full quality). This would mean that, even given these generous assumptions, treatment would be evaluated at a cost of £150,000 per QALY, well over the current threshold of £30,000 per QALY.

Alternatively, we could try to assess, for example, what chance of survival would have been high enough for a trial of treatment to have been cost-effective for Charlie Gard. We could calculate this based on the costs of 3 months of intensive care and we could assume, if the treatment were successful, that Charlie would survive for 5 to 10 years. The probability threshold for providing treatment would be ~50%–100%.[d] In other words, using these assumptions, there would have to have been a more than 50% chance of treatment working for it to be cost-effective enough to provide it within the public health system in the UK. If it was expected that Charlie would have significantly reduced quality of life, even in the best-case scenario of treatment being successful (and if this is thought to be relevant to take into account), the probability threshold would rise. For example, if it was thought that Charlie were likely to still be severely impaired (with a value for quality of life lower than 0.4), 3 months of intensive care treatment would not fall within the NHS cost-effectiveness threshold, even if it had a 100% chance of working.

This analysis is obviously highly simplified. It includes assumptions that might be questioned (though we have erred on the side of generosity). The aim here is not to analyse in detail the cost-effectiveness of treatment for Charlie. Rather, it is to make three points:

1. Cost-effectiveness thresholds could be used to estimate when it would and would not be reasonable to provide treatment in a public healthcare system. They could provide an answer to the difficult question of how high a chance of survival needs to be to provide treatment. For example, elsewhere, in a more general analysis of cost limits to treatment in intensive care, we estimated that it would be cost-effective to provide 20 days of intensive care to an adult with a chance of survival of >9% (assuming full quality of life).[38] It would be cost-effective to provide a highly expensive form of life support (extracorporeal membrane oxygenation; ECMO) to a newborn with a more than 17% chance of survival.[39]

2. If we use thresholds like this, the argument against providing intensive care treatment in some cases becomes clearer. In the UK, it is not uncommon for expensive new treatments (for example, cancer drugs) to be declined because they fall outside the cost-effectiveness threshold. As one example, the breast cancer drug Kadcyla is thought to extend life by an average of 9 months at an annual cost of £90,000. It was not approved by the UK NHS treatment appraisal body because of its high cost.[e] It would seem, on the face of it, unfair

---

[d]Cost-effectiveness = cost of treatment / effect. The effect of treatment could be estimated by multiplying the chance of survival by the number of QALY obtained. Transforming this equation, the probability threshold (the minimum chance of survival for treatment to be cost-effective, P_T) = cost of treatment / (cost-effectiveness threshold × quality × duration of survival). Calculation based on an estimated cost of treatment of £150,000, a cost-effectiveness threshold of £30,000, quality of life of 1, and survival duration of 5–10 years.

[e]The estimated cost/QALY of Kadcyla was ~£160,000.[40] NICE eventually reconsidered this decision in June 2017 after re-analyzing data, and after negotiating a lower price for the drug.

to refuse to fund treatment for some patients because that would not be cost-effective, but then to provide treatment (intensive care) to other patients that may be even more costly and less effective.

3. Clarifying how resource constraints might be applied to cases like that of Charlie Gard highlights some of the competing values that are at stake in deciding how limited resources should be allocated. We will return to this later.

Modified triage

We noted earlier that it is hard to apply a triage model to decisions about providing treatment in intensive care because patients don't arrive needing treatment at the same time. In our triage example, it was relatively clear that doctors should treat infant B (with a 94% chance of survival) rather an infant A (with a 3% chance of survival). However, if infant A is referred alone for treatment, doctors may embark on treatment and then find that they have no intensive care bed when the infant with better chances needs treatment.

One way of resolving this problem would be to use a modified form of triage. In a paper in 1992, Robert Truog proposed that triage-style comparisons for patients needing a scarce life-saving treatment could be made sequentially. New patients would be compared with patients already receiving treatment.[41] For example:

Infant A has a genetic disorder causing severe lung disease. They were commenced on treatment in intensive care yesterday. The estimated chance of survival with treatment is less than 3%.

Infant B has severe lung problems due to a temporary disorder arising at birth. They have just been referred for treatment, and it is estimated that their chance of survival with intensive care is as high as 94%.

If there are no intensive care beds available, and no way to provide treatment for both patients, the suggestion is that treatment could be withdrawn from the first patient to make it available for the second.

There are different ways that this sort of modified triage could work. A new patient needing treatment (when there is no bed available) could be compared with the last patient who was admitted (this would give us a comparison that is analogous to the two patients arriving at the same time). Alternatively, the new patient could be compared to the patient in the ICU who has the worst chance of survival. (That would give the new patient the best chance of receiving treatment, while also meaning that the ICU saves the largest number of lives.) Or we might compare the new patient with whichever patient in the ICU has received treatment for the longest. (That would even out the share of intensive care between different patients.)[f]

One advantage of modified triage is that it avoids situations where doctors refuse to treat patients (who could benefit from treatment) in a desire to save an intensive care bed for a potential future patient (who would benefit more). It would reduce the chances of patients missing out on a chance of intensive care. It may also allow extra information to be gathered that will allow more accurate estimates of a patient's chance of survival.

Yet, one challenge for modified triage is that it requires doctors to be prepared to withdraw treatment from one patient to make it available to another patient. Many health professionals

---

[f]One other possibility, sometimes labelled 'reverse triage', would seek to discharge from the intensive care unit the most stable patient, in order to make way for the new patient needing treatment.

find it psychologically more difficult to stop a treatment than to decide not to start a treatment.[42] People, including doctors, intuitively believe there is a morally relevant distinction between actions and omissions, though philosophically this is very difficult to defend.[43]

Our own experience of working with and teaching doctors in intensive care suggests that, while many would find it straightforward in the triage case to treat infant B rather than infant A, relatively few would be prepared in the modified triage case to stop treatment in infant A in order to provide it to infant B.

But is there actually an ethical difference between stopping (withdrawing) treatment and not starting (withholding) treatment? Here are three reasons why (when all other factors are the same) there is not an ethical difference:

1. **The outcome is the same.** If doctors decide not to provide life-saving treatment to a patient with a low chance of survival, or if they decide to stop providing a life-saving treatment to a patient with the same low chance of survival, the patient will die. That is a bad thing to happen. But it is equally bad for the patient to die whether or not they have received treatment (unless the treatment caused them to suffer).

2. **The doctors' intention is the same.** The aim of the intensive care doctors is to help patients and save lives. When they cannot treat everyone, they aim to make a fair decision and do the most good with treatment. That aim is the same, whether they are performing triage or modified triage.

3. **It is equally fair (or unfair).** If we think that it is fair to provide treatment to the infant with better chances (infant B) in the triage case, it seems equally fair to provide treatment to infant B in modified triage. (If we think that it is unfair to deny treatment to the infant with low chance of survival, it would surely be just as unfair to take away treatment.)

Modified triage seems highly relevant to the Charlie Gard case. We do not know if there were other patients needing treatment at the time when he was first admitted to the ICU. However, by the time that he had been in the ICU for several months, it is highly likely that there would have been multiple other patients needing treatment at Great Ormond Street. By that point in time, there was enough information about Charlie's condition and outlook that, whether or not we believe that it would or could benefit him to have treatment continued, it is very clear that other children needing treatment in intensive care would have better chances of survival and would benefit more. (Of course, such an argument would not have precluded Charlie being taken to the US for treatment.)

Fairness and discrimination

If we provide intensive care to patients with a very poor prognosis, that may mean that other patients (who would benefit more) aren't able to receive treatment. That is a serious problem for healthcare systems with limited resources. It means that the public healthcare system is not able to benefit patients as much as it could. On the other hand, if some patients are denied intensive care because of lack of resources, that seems to generate a different sort of problem. If doctors choose to treat some patients (with better outlook) but not others, that might seem to be a form of discrimination. It seems to conflict with the ideal of equal access to treatment and is potentially unfair.

The first point to make here is that any time that doctors or health systems make decisions about who to treat they are 'discriminating'. The word can be used to refer to any process of identifying and acting on differences. If those differences are ethically relevant, discrimination can be justified. So, for example, choosing to treat a sicker patient first in the emergency department is a form of discrimination. Some people have to wait longer before being seen. But it is not unfair discrimination. What would be unfair, though, is to preferentially treat patients in the emergency department based on ethically irrelevant characteristics (e.g., race, gender, political or religious views). Whether discrimination is ethically problematic depends on what characteristics are used and whether they are ethically relevant or not.

What about disability? Would it be unfair discrimination to deny a patient treatment on the basis of a disability? Earlier in this chapter we imagined an intensive care triage case. We suggested that it would be justified, in that case, to provide the last intensive care bed to the patient who would benefit more from treatment – the one with a better chance of survival (rather than tossing a coin to choose). That is discrimination, but it isn't necessarily unfair discrimination, even though we are choosing not to provide treatment to the infant with a genetic condition (a form of disability), meaning that they have very low chance of survival.

There are different ways in which an underlying condition might mean that patients benefit more or less from treatment. Here are several different possibilities:

A. Cost of treatment. A child might have an underlying health condition that means that it would be more expensive to treat them.

B. Duration of treatment. A child's health condition means that treatment (for example, intensive care) would be required for a longer period.

C. Chance of survival. A child's health condition means that they have a reduced chance of surviving.

D. Chance of improvement with treatment (for a non–life-saving treatment). A child's health condition means that they have a lower probability that treatment will help them.

E. Magnitude of improvement with treatment (for a non–life-saving treatment). A child's health condition means that treatment will help them by a smaller degree.

F. Duration of survival. A child's health condition means that they are expected to live for a shorter time.

G. Quality of life. A child's underlying health condition means that they will have a reduced quality of life.

We have separated these out, though in a real case, a child's health condition might reduce their benefit from treatment in several ways. In a more complex case, they might be better in some ways and worse in others.

If we are reflecting on whether it would be unfair discrimination to deny a child life-saving treatment, it may depend on which of these reasons is the basis for not providing treatment. It may be that some of them are more fair or unfair than others. For example, some people might feel that it would not be unfair discrimination in the triage case to treat a patient with a higher chance of survival, but that it would be unfair to treat a patient with a higher expected quality of life.

Here is one reason for thinking that some of these reasons are more unfair than others. At the start of this chapter, we gave the analogy of dividing up a chocolate cake. It would be unfair for some people to have an extra-large slice of cake (or an extra slice) if that meant that others would receive less (or that fewer people would get a slice). Some of the reasons given above are like the extra-large slice. For example, if treatment would be more expensive (A), that would potentially mean that there are less funds available to help other patients. It means that a smaller number of people are able to be treated.

The same would apply to someone needing a longer duration of a scarce treatment like intensive care (B). If an ICU is often at capacity (i.e., there are no spare beds), and one patient requires intensive care for twice as long as other patients, that means that fewer patients are able to be admitted to the ICU. That may mean that, when thinking about allocation of scarce intensive care beds, we should be particularly concerned about patients who require prolonged treatment.

These are what we could call 'different number' cases,[g] as they mean that it is possible to treat more or fewer patients. If doctors are in a position to help a larger group of patients (and all patients have an equal claim to treatment), it is not unfair to discriminate.

But other reasons given earlier aren't like the large slice of cake. If there are two patients needing intensive care, and one has a lower quality of life than the other, a decision to treat one rather than the other is a 'same number' case. This is like someone choosing who will get a (standard-sized) slice of cake, and deciding to give it to Fred rather than Freya because they believe that Fred is hungrier. Reasons E (magnitude of improvement), F (duration of survival) and G (quality of life) all seem to be 'same number' cases. We might have much more concern for fairness or equality in cases like this.

What about situations where one patient has a lower chance of survival (or a lower chance of improvement) (reasons C and D from the list)? Do these count as 'same number' or as 'different number' cases? If doctors decide to preferentially allocate treatment to patients who have a higher chance of survival, that will mean that they treat the same number of patients. Some people might view these as 'same number' cases and claim that it would be unfair to give preference to the patient with a higher chance of survival. Others might point out that ICUs that give priority to patients with higher survival chances will save the life of a larger number of patients. So, in a sense, this could also be viewed as a 'different number' case. Returning to our cake analogy, imagine that we have only one slice of cake and two people to choose from. We do not know if they will like this cake, but one of them is fussy and there is only a small chance that they will like this cake. We know the other person likes almost all cakes, and there is a high chance they will enjoy the cake. Would it be fair to give the slice to the person who is highly likely to enjoy it? Or should we toss a coin? There are different reasonable views about that question.

Some of the reasons given for deciding which patient to treat are more controversial than others. Some of them are harder to estimate or quantify. In particular, deciding not to provide life-saving treatment because a patient has reduced expected quality of life might be thought to be unjustified because it is unfair. We might also be particularly cautious about rationing treatment on the basis of quality of life because this is so difficult to measure or quantify. As we noted in Chapter 3, there are different reasonable views about how we should evaluate quality of life and about how much some disabling conditions reduce quality of life. However, we do not need to definitively answer that question here. Even if we reject the use of quality of life to determine whether or not to provide intensive care, there are other reasons that seem important and relevant to consider for limited resources. Providing prolonged duration of treatment or highly expensive treatment to one patient, where that would lead to other patients being harmed, seems unfair.

Withholding life-saving treatment from a child because of limited resources may be more or less unfair depending on the reason for denying treatment. It may also be a question of degree. If we imagine a variant of the triage case, where a doctor had to choose between treating a child with normal intelligence and a child with a mild disability (for example, a learning difficulty), it might seem unfair to simply choose the child with higher intelligence. (If forced to choose, perhaps the doctor should simply choose whichever child arrived first or toss a coin.) But if the difference between patients was much greater, it seems less and less unfair. If there were a choice between providing life-saving treatment to a child who will have a normal life and a child who

---

[g]In discussing the ethics of population, Derek Parfit famously distinguished between 'same-number' and 'different-number' cases.[44] He argued that cases in which more or fewer people exist raised a distinct set of ethical considerations from cases where the same number of people exist. The context here is different. It is not whether different numbers of people exist, instead whether different numbers of people will have their life saved.

is permanently unconscious, it would certainly be justified to choose to save the first child. Some people might feel that the latter choice is clear because it would be futile to provide intensive care to a child who is permanently unconscious. However, in Chapter 2 we pointed out the difficulty of determining or defining futility (particularly when it comes to quality of life). We can't rely on futility to help us allocate resources.

Permanent unconsciousness is an example of extreme disability or impairment in quality of life, but similar arguments would apply to profound cognitive impairment. Most people do consider a very reduced quality or length of survival to be a relevant factor,[25] and using such factors is supported by several moral theories, such as utilitarianism or contractualism.[45,46]

How does this help us with allocating the scarce resource of intensive care? We have described two different ethical values that are important in how we allocate limited health resources. One of these is a desire to be fair and to give patients equal consideration. The other is a desire to do the most good from our healthcare system. Our allocation process needs to balance these different values.

We described a potential way to work out when treatment in intensive care would not be cost-effective (and consequently, when providing treatment would potentially harm other patients). We showed that cost-effectiveness could identify a probability threshold – the lowest chance of survival when it would potentially be cost-effective to provide intensive care. A similar analysis could be done to assess thresholds for other variables – for example, based on the highest cost of treatment or duration of intensive care, the shortest predicted length of survival or the lowest quality of life.

Those answers to the question of allocating treatment are based only on generating the most health benefit from intensive care. However, if we are wishing to balance benefit with equality or fairness, we should lower the threshold (i.e., be more generous in providing treatment). It is beyond the scope of this book to analyse how exactly decision makers might try to reach the right compromise between equality and benefit; however, some basic principles may be useful.

How far we go depends on how much weight we place on the value of equality. For example, we suggested earlier that, based on cost-effectiveness, ECMO might be an option for infants with a more than 17% chance of survival. However, we could lower this threshold because of concern for equality and offer ECMO to infants with a more than 10% chance of survival, but not, say, a 1% chance of survival. If we are considering quality of life and provision of intensive care, we may want to give particular weight to fairness (this would also give acknowledgment to the variation in reasonable views about acceptable quality of life). That may mean only withholding treatment in cases where quality of life is markedly reduced (and perhaps where there is genuine uncertainty whether treatment would overall be a benefit).[47]

One way of giving greater weight to fairness and equality than to overall benefit would be to draw on the concept of 'cost equivalence' in allocation of resources. We have argued elsewhere that, where patients (or parents) are requesting nonstandard medical treatment, one fair approach would be to allow access to treatment as long as it is equivalent in cost to the standard treatment. This would allow patients to access treatments that they desire, but not at the expense of other patients. It might mean, in the case of providing intensive care treatment, that patients could access treatment even if the benefit (in terms of chance of success, duration of survival or quality of life) is small but could not access more expensive or more prolonged treatment. In Chapter 8 we will apply this sort of approach to avoiding prolonged treatment in intensive care through the use of time-limited trials of treatment.

Conclusion

In the last chapter we outlined some of the challenges and uncertainties involved in determining whether or not treatment would be in a child's best interests. There is considerable difficulty in weighing up the benefits and harms of treatment, in assessing quality of life and in evaluating treatments with small chances of working. We suggested a preliminary conclusion in that chapter that would accommodate pluralism about interests and uncertainty. Given uncertainty about best interests and a life worth living, we should generally err on the side of accepting parents' views. Where there is a possibility (based upon a reasonable evaluation of the facts) that treatment would be beneficial, it would be permissible for treatment to be provided or continued.

However, in this chapter we have discussed some competing considerations that might count against providing possibly beneficial treatment. Even if treatment would potentially be in a child's best interests, there may be situations (particularly where treatment is expensive and/or limited in availability) where it should not be provided, on the basis of distributive justice. What level of certainty should we adopt for these judgments? If we are trying to decide how to allocate our limited healthcare resources, we cannot always be certain that treatment will work and will constitute good value for money. Yet, if we use our limited resources to provide treatment that is only *possibly* of benefit, it is inevitable that, in many situations, treatment will be of no help or will do more harm than good. It seems that, where resources are scarce, it would be prudent to provide treatment that is *probably* of overall benefit and probably falls within the affordability limits of the health system. For those health systems that employ cost-effectiveness analysis, treatment in intensive care (as other forms of treatment) should be provided if it is *likely* to be cost-effective. We have outlined how this might be applied.

Here is our own view of factors that ought to be considered to maximise the number of people who benefit from limited resources like intensive care. Treatment should be preferentially provided to those with:

   A. Lower cost of treatment.
   B. Shorter duration of treatment.
   C. Higher chance of survival.

When there is a particularly low value for the following factors, these should potentially reduce a patient's priority for treatment:

   A. Lower probability of improvement with treatment (for a non–life-saving treatment).
   B. Shorter duration of survival.
   C. Lower quality of life.

What about health systems that do not apply cost-effectiveness thresholds (such as private systems)? Because intensive care beds are a scarce resource, there are reasons to limit provision of treatment even in such health systems. One way of applying limits would be to use modified triage once the unit reached capacity. Another way might be to provide treatment for a maximum length of time (beyond which continued treatment would probably lead to other patients being denied care). How long treatment should be provided would depend upon the capacity of an ICU (how often it was full and having to turn patients away) and the usual length of stay. The expectation would be that, once patients had received a maximum duration of therapy, they would be transferred elsewhere (to an alternative facility with greater capacity prepared to take them), or treatment would be withdrawn.

As we have argued, it is in many ways ethically easier and more justifiable to limit potentially life-saving medical treatment on the basis of distributive justice and fair allocation of resources than on the grounds that it will not benefit the patient (is not in his or her interests). In general, given value pluralism and rejection of medical paternalism, we are on more defensible territory discussing justice than what is in another person's best interests. Of course, decisions about interests have to be made, and require further ethical work, but questions of limits to treatment can be more tractably addressed from the perspective of justice. While we have used the example of intensive care, our arguments apply to any medical resource or treatment, such as surgery, drugs or even the time of personnel.

We have focused on allocation of existing health resources. There is a further question about how much should be spent on healthcare compared with other priorities. Some of the difficulties that doctors face in deciding whether or not to provide treatment might be reduced if more funding were allocated to healthcare rather than other national projects or priorities.

However, even in the wealthiest countries with the most well-funded health systems, there will still be a limit to resources, and questions of distributive justice will still need to be addressed.

We will return in Chapter 8 to thinking about how, in practice, societies should derive thresholds for treatment, and how they should assess whether thresholds have been reached for individual patients. Before we do that, though, we need to focus on another question – how treatments are evaluated (how evidence is collected and appraised). Furthermore, we need to consider how or when treatments might be provided that have only had an incomplete evaluation, i.e., experimental treatment. For experimental treatments, it is, by definition, unclear whether or not they are of benefit. How should we approach the question of whether or when they should be available?

References

1. *Great Ormond Street Hospital v Yates & Ors* [2017] EWHC 972 (Fam) (11 April 2017) para 81.
2. https://www.rushlimbaugh.com/daily/2017/07/10/exclusive-vice-president-mike-pence-calls-the-show/
3. Wilkinson, D. & Savulescu, J. (2012) A costly separation between withdrawing and withholding treatment in intensive care. *Bioethics*, 26, 32-48.
4. Noyes, J., Godfrey, C. & Beecham, J. (2006) Resource use and service costs for ventilator-dependent children and young people in the UK. *Health & social care in the community*, 14, 508-22.
5. Government statistical service. (2017). '*Monthly critical care beds and cancelled urgent operations data, England March 2017.*' From <https://www.england.nhs.uk/statistics/wp-content/uploads/sites/2/2016/05/March-17-Monthly-SitRep-SPN.pdf>.
6. Faculty of Intensive Care Medicine & Intensive Care Society. (2015). '*Guidelines for the provision of intensive care services.*' In G. Masterson and S. Baudouin (Eds.). From <https://www.ics.ac.uk/ICS/guidelines-and-standards.aspx>.
7. https://www.england.nhs.uk/statistics/wp-content/uploads/sites/2/2016/05/MSitRep-March-2017-1abF7.xls
8. Menzel, P. T. (2003) How compatible are liberty and equality in structuring a health care system? *J Med Philos*, 28, 281-306.
9. *Professor Robert Truog. Personal correspondence.*
10. Truog, R. D. (2017) The United Kingdom Sets Limits on Experimental Treatments: The Case of Charlie Gard. *JAMA*, 318, 1001-1002.
11. Keehan, S. P., Stone, D. A., Poisal, J. A., Cuckler, G. A., Sisko, A. M., Smith, S. D., et al. (2017) National Health Expenditure Projections, 2016-25: Price Increases, Aging Push Sector To 20 Percent Of Economy. *Health Aff (Millwood)*, 36, 553-563.
12. Ham, C. (1999b) Tragic choices in health care: lessons from the child B case. *BMJ*, 319, 1258-61.
13. *R. v Cambridge Health Authority [1995] EWCA Civ 49.*
14. Ham, C. (1999b) Tragic choices in health care: lessons from the child B case. *BMJ*, 319, 1258-61.
15. Foster, C. (2007) Simple rationality? The law of healthcare resource allocation in England. *J Med Ethics*, 33, 404-7.
16. Ham, C. (1999a) The role of doctors, patients and managers in priority setting decisions: lessons from the 'Child B' case. *Health Expect*, 2, 61-68.
17. *Portsmouth NHS Trust v Wyatt* [2005] 1 F.L.R. 21.
18. Laurance, J. (1998) Child B: the truth about her last days. *Independent*. Accessed from <http://www.independent.co.uk/life-style/child-b-the-truth-about-her-last-days-1159951.html>.
19. Ham, C. (1999a) The role of doctors, patients and managers in priority setting decisions: lessons from the 'Child B' case. *Health Expect*, 2, 61-68.

20. Chandler, M. (2017) Charlie Gard parents hit £1.2m fundraising target for sick baby's pioneering US treatment. *Evening Standard*. Accessed from <https://www.standard.co.uk/news/london/charlie-gard-parents-hit-12m-fundraising-target-for-sick-babys-pioneering-us-treatment-a3505106.html>.
21. https://www.whatdotheyknow.com/request/cost_of_legal_action_in_high_cou
22. http://www.gosh.nhs.uk/about-us/our-corporate-information/how-we-spend/annual-accounts
23. (2017b). 'Critical Care Bed Capacity and Urgent Operations Cancelled 2017-18 Data.' From <https://www.england.nhs.uk/statistics/statistical-work-areas/critical-care-capacity/critical-care-bed-capacity-and-urgent-operations-cancelled-2017-18-data/>.
24. Aacharya, R. P., Gastmans, C. & Denier, Y. (2011) Emergency department triage: an ethical analysis. *BMC emergency medicine*, 11, 16.
25. Arora, C., Savulescu, J., Maslen, H., Selgelid, M. & Wilkinson, D. (2016) The Intensive Care Lifeboat: a survey of lay attitudes to rationing dilemmas in neonatal intensive care. *BMC Med Ethics*, 17, 69.
26. Teres, D. (1993) Civilian triage in the intensive care unit: the ritual of the last bed. *Crit Care Med*, 21, 598-606.
27. Simoens, S. (2009) Health economic assessment: a methodological primer. *Int J Environ Res Public Health*, 6, 2950-66, Cleemput, I., Neyt, M., Thiry, N., De Laet, C. & Leys, M. (2011) Using threshold values for cost per quality-adjusted life-year gained in healthcare decisions. *Int J Technol Assess Health Care*, 27, 71-6.
28. Neumann, P. J., Cohen, J. T. & Weinstein, M. C. (2014) Updating cost-effectiveness—the curious resilience of the $50,000-per-QALY threshold. *N Engl J Med*, 371, 796-797.
29. Grosse, S. D. (2008) Assessing cost-effectiveness in healthcare: history of the $50,000 per QALY threshold. *Expert Rev Pharmacoecon Outcomes Res*, 8, 165-78.
30. Dubois, R. W. (2016) Cost-effectiveness thresholds in the USA: are they coming? Are they already here? *J Comp Eff Res*, 5, 9-11.
31. Sullivan, S. D., Yeung, K., Vogeler, C., Ramsey, S. D., Wong, E., Murphy, C. O., et al. (2015) Design, implementation, and first-year outcomes of a value-based drug formulary. *J Manag Care Spec Pharm*, 21, 269-75.
32. Harris, J. (1987) QALYfying the value of life. *J Med Ethics*, 13, 117-23.
33. Singer, P., McKie, J., Kuhse, H. & Richardson, J. (1995) Double jeopardy and the use of QALYs in health care allocation. *J Med Ethics*. 21, 144-50.
34. Nord, E., Daniels, N. & Kamlet, M. (2009) QALYs: some challenges. *Value Health*, 12 Suppl 1, S10-5.
35. McMillan, J. & Hope, T. (2010) Balancing principles, QALYs, and the straw men of resource allocation. *Am J Bioethics*, 10, 48-50.
36. Bognar, G. & Hirose, I. (2014) *The ethics of health care rationing : an introduction*. Abingdon, Oxon, Routledge.
37. (2017c) *Charlie Gard has 10% chance of improvement, US doctor claims. BBC online*. Accessed from <http://www.bbc.co.uk/news/uk-england-london-40593286>.
38. Wilkinson, D., Petrou, S. & Savulescu, J. (2018) Expensive care? Resource-based thresholds for potentially inappropriate treatment in intensive care. *Monash Bioeth Rev* https://doi.org/10.1007/s40592-017-0075-5.
39. Wilkinson, D., Petrou, S. & Savulescu, J. (2018) Rationing potentially inappropriate treatment in newborn intensive care in developed countries. *Semin Fetal Neonatal Med* 23, 52-58.
40. National Institute for Health and Care Excellence. (2014). '*Pressure grows on Roche to lower breast cancer drug price*'. From <https://www.nice.org.uk/news/article/pressure-grows-on-roche-to-lower-breast-cancer-drug-price>.
41. Truog, R. D. (1992) Triage in the ICU. *Hastings Cent Rep*, 22, 13-17.
42. Wilkinson, D. & Savulescu, J. (2012) A costly separation between withdrawing and withholding treatment in intensive care. *Bioethics*, 26, 32-48.
43. Rachels, J. (1975) Active and passive euthanasia. *N Engl J Med*, 292, 78-80.
44. Parfit, D. (1982) Future generations: further problems. *Philos Public Aff*, 11, 113-172.
45. Savulescu, J. (2001) Resources, Down's syndrome, and cardiac surgery. *BMJ*, 322, 875-6.
46. Scanlon, T. (1998) *What we owe to each other*. Cambridge, Mass.; London, Belknap.
47. Wilkinson, D. & Savulescu, J. (forthcoming) Prioritisation and parity: which disabled infants should be candidates for scarce life-saving treatment. In A. Cureton and D. Wasserman (Eds.) *Oxford Handbook of Philosophy and Disability*. Oxford University Press.

CHAPTER 5

Research

> 'Science is out of the reach of morals, for her eyes are fixed upon eternal truths.'
>
> **The Critic as Artist, Oscar Wilde**

> '[A]ll life is an experiment. Every year if not every day we have to wager our salvation upon some prophecy based upon imperfect knowledge.'
>
> JUSTICE HOLMES, 1919[1]

> 'Charlie suffers from the RRM2B mutation of MDDS. No one in the world has ever treated this form of MDDS with nucleoside therapy.... I dare say that medical science may benefit, objectively, from the experiment, but experimentation cannot be in Charlie's best interests unless there is a prospect of benefit for him.'
>
> JUSTICE FRANCIS, APRIL 11[2]

As famously described by Justice Holmes almost a century ago, uncertainty affects all aspects of life. How should we decide when that uncertainty is too great? Justice Francis' logic in denying Charlie Gard access to experimental treatment appears at first sight to be convincing and objective. However, science is not (despite the claims of Oscar Wilde's protagonist Gilbert) beyond the reach of morals. On the contrary, embedded in these seemingly factual claims are value judgments that are highly contested. In this chapter, we explore the relationship between science, research and values. We will outline some of the ethical principles that govern when research can take place and when it must not take place. We will identify the challenge in determining how much harm is low enough to allow research in noncompetent patients, when the evidence is sufficient that trials must cease, when a patient is too sick to participate in a trial and when there is enough expert support of an innovative treatment. There are a range of different reasonable views about many of these questions.

Science and ethics

One of the greatest human achievements is science. Scientific method has revolutionised the world and life. Cars, refrigerators, electricity, computers and, of course, modern medicine all mean humans have better lives than ever before. Science has proven itself as the preeminent way of understanding ourselves and the world around us. The power of science is manifested in its ability to say how the world will change according to scientific laws. It can, in this sense, predict the future.

Science tells us facts. It refers to how things are, were, will be, could be, might be. It tells us how we can change the world around us. Ethics, in contrast, is a different form of knowledge and enquiry. Ethics is about values or norms. It is about how we or the world around us should be, ought to be, must be. It is about good and bad, right and wrong. When we use normative language like 'ought', 'should', 'good', 'desirable', 'right', 'virtuous', 'must', we are in the province of ethics.

71

David Hume famously pointed out that an 'ought' (a value judgment) can never be derived directly from an 'is' (a factual statement). This is sometimes called the 'naturalistic fallacy'.

> 'In every system of morality, … the author proceeds for sometime in the ordinary way of reasoning, and establishes the being of a God, or makes observations concerning human affairs; when of a sudden I am surprised to find, that instead of the usual copulations of propositions, is, and is not, I meet with no proposition that is not connected with an ought, or an ought not. The change is imperceptible; but is, of the last consequence. For as this ought and ought not expresses some new relation or affirmation, 'tis necessary that it should be observed and explained; and at the same time that a reason should be given, for what seems altogether inconceivable, how this new relation can be a deduction from others, which are entirely different from it.'[3]

Every decision to act, including a decision to experiment, involves values in the form of a goal. The choice to experiment on some toxin could derive from the value of curing disease, or from the aim of wiping out a population with a bioweapon. And every action requires facts about the world to understand which course of action is most likely to realise a particular value. Thus, science needs ethics, and ethics needs science. We need ethics to supply the value or goals – what is worth achieving – and we need science to tell us how to achieve those goals.

Ethics and science are related in other ways. Ethics places constraints on how scientific research should be conducted. In Nazi Germany, doctors and scientists performed lethal and horrific experiments on Jews and other minorities, such as exposing them to freezing water to see how long it took to die. They conducted gruesome surgeries on twins, gave people infectious diseases and committed other atrocious crimes. Many of these experiments were devised to develop medical treatments to support injured or ill German soldiers.

These appalling experiments, amongst other atrocities, led to the first internationally agreed guidelines on research involving people, the Nuremberg Code (1946), which was incorporated by the medical profession into the Declaration of Helsinki in 1964.

The importance of research

There is a moral imperative to perform good research and not unnecessarily impede it. To delay by one year the development of a treatment that cures a lethal disease that kills 100,000 people per year is to be responsible for the deaths of those 100,000 people, even if you never see them.[4] Ethics committees and laws that obstruct good research are themselves unethical.[5]

The point of research is to gain knowledge. It is not necessarily to benefit the patients or people who take part, though they may derive benefit. Rather, the main point of medical research is to gain knowledge to benefit all patients, those now and in the future. As the risk posed to human participants increases, there must be a greater prospect of benefit either to participants or to people in the future. The risks must be proportionate to the potential gains. These are ethical evaluations.

The point of research is also to gather evidence. Evidence can come from many sources. For example, we can gather evidence from our senses, or by observation. However, we are prone to many psychological and perceptual biases.[6] For this reason, more structured experiments are conducted to control for bias and for multiple variables that might influence an outcome. The paradigm example is the randomised placebo-controlled clinical trial.

Sometimes you will hear of 'levels of evidence' or quality of evidence. This reflects the degree of scientific rigour in clinical research. Studies range from randomised controlled trials (highest level of evidence), to cohort studies, to case-control studies to expert opinions (lowest).

The more significant a problem, or the larger the numbers of people affected, the higher the level of evidence required. As an individual, you might choose a treatment that is probably (just more than 50/50 chance) better than an alternative. However, when a drug must be administered to very large numbers of people, risking significant side effects and costing significant amounts of money, then much higher levels of confidence are required. How much evidence is 'enough', however, is an ethical question, as we will see later. The level of evidence and justification for action that is required depends on the situation and context. Low levels can be sufficient to justify action where only a single person or small group of individuals are affected.

Ethical principles in research

CONSENT

One feature of research ethics which we will not consider in detail is the requirement to obtain consent. The most famous and influential code governing research is The Declaration of Helsinki, developed by the World Medical Association. In paragraph 26, the Declaration states that:

'... the physician or another appropriately qualified individual must then seek the potential subject's freely-given informed consent, preferably in writing.'[7]

Some guidelines, and the Mental Capacity Act (2005),[8] do allow research with participants lacking capacity to consent to the research but only if the risk of harm is very low and, in most guidelines, only if consent is given by a proxy, such as a parent. That raises the question of what counts as a very low risk of harm, as we will describe later.

SCIENTIFIC JUSTIFICATION: VALIDITY AND NECESSITY

The Declaration of Helsinki (paragraph 21) emphasises the importance of research conforming to 'generally accepted scientific principles'.[7] Research that is scientifically flawed is unethical because it will not benefit people in the future and so any risk of harm to participants cannot be justified. It may harm people in the future because the results are misleading or because it uses up resources which could be directed to potentially beneficial research.

Research that fails to take account of existing evidence exposes participants to risk unnecessarily.[7] For this reason, a systematic review of the literature is necessary prior to conducting any scientific research. The failure to conduct a systematic review of the literature can be lethal. In the case of healthy volunteer Ellen Roche, researchers failed to identify the risks of hexamethonium known from previous research, resulting in her death in an asthma study.[9]

Another issue in establishing scientific validity is whether the hypothesis to be tested is sufficiently plausible. This will often depend on existing research and knowledge, and whether there is a reasonable inference to the hypothesis. For example, in the case of Charlie Gard, Professor Hirano hypothesised that nucleoside replacement therapy might have an effect on Charlie's form of mitochondrial DNA depletion syndrome (MDDS). This was based on experience of nucleoside replacement therapy having an effect in the milder *TK2* deficiency, some evidence that nucleoside replacement therapy crossed the blood-brain barrier and evidence of effect in cultured human cells with *RR2MB* deficiency.

Because nucleoside replacement therapy had never been tried in the *RR2MB*-related form of MDDS, it would be experimental. Was it a reasonable experiment? In this case, both Hirano and Charlie's parents hoped it would have some beneficial effect for Charlie, as well as generating knowledge. The doctors and the judge, however, believed it was 'futile'. As we discussed in Chapter 2, determining that a chance of success is sufficiently low that it is futile involves value judgments.

EXPERIMENTATION

If the chances were low, but not zero, whether such an experiment would be justified would then turn on the benefits and burdens of the experiment to Charlie.

What is clear is that whether the benefits to Charlie outweigh the burdens is an ethical, not scientific, judgment.

In the case of Charlie Gard, Judge Francis accepted that providing the treatment might benefit others by generating valuable scientific information, however, he did not believe that it would benefit Charlie to receive experimental treatment.[2] Ethically, whether an experiment could be done for knowledge's sake, without prospect of benefit, depends at least in part in the harm it causes. Such benefits ought to be included if the harms are reasonable. Again, that takes us back to the question of whether the harms to Charlie were reasonable.

In a different, hypothetical, research project, one of us has argued that research might be ethical in a dying patient if the harms are minimal and the benefit of the knowledge significant. Consider first the case of a competent person.

> 'Consider a controversial research proposal: lethal research. Research which will inevitably kill a human being is not permitted under any research code. But should such research in principle ever be approved? … Consider a person in a jurisdiction that permits voluntary euthanasia. Imagine that this person, John, has terminal liver cancer and wishes to die now rather than suffering and dying in the further future. This is an entirely reasonable wish. But let us assume also that John has an altruistic streak—he would like some good to come of his death. He volunteers for a highly risky experiment. Perhaps it is some new phase I trial or some new intracranial device implantation or novel surgical procedure. Or perhaps he wishes to contribute to knowledge of severe infections, like Ebola, and would participate in a lethal challenge study.
> John knows he will fall asleep, just as he would with conventional euthanasia, and never wake up. But in the interval between him falling asleep and him finally dying, he will contribute to science. He will, in effect, have donated his body to science. Instead of no good coming from his death, some good would come of it. We could call this voluntary research euthanasia (VRE).'[10]

In this case, a competent person consents to take part in research when he or she will no longer be conscious. Young children cannot consent to taking part in research. They are not likely to understand the value of research for other people or have a desire to take part in such research. But nonetheless, if a baby were unconscious and were certainly going to die, but a research procedure could be done purely to gain knowledge before that baby died, it might be justifiable. What matters is the baby's suffering, and if suffering is not present, then scientific research that could potentially lead to breakthroughs could be justified. We might feel that is because everyone (even babies) has an innate altruistic interest – in promoting the wellbeing of others. Then perhaps it is 'in' the child's interest. Or perhaps we would justify it through concern for the parents' interests and their decision to see something good come from the death of their child. Or perhaps we justify this because of concern for the interests of wider society (where it isn't against the interests of the child).

Very similar issues arise when organ donation is contemplated for young children. Sometimes life support is continued or extra treatments are provided while preparations are made for organ donation. This is not directly for the benefit of the child, but as long as the harms are negligible, it is usually thought to be justified.[11]

Many people will object that this opens the door to research on unconscious and brain-dead people and babies. This is true. Whether such research can be justified will depend on the case and context. In the case of Charlie Gard, if Charlie Gard were placed under anaesthesia, perhaps such an experiment, purely for knowledge's sake, could have been justified. It seems likely his parents would have consented.

MINIMAL HARMS

The Declaration of Helsinki cites the second principle of the Declaration of Geneva: 'The health and well-being of my patient will be my first consideration'[12] and the International Code of Medical Ethics: 'A physician shall act in the patient's best interest when providing medical care'.[13] All ethical codes and principles, just like laws, must be interpreted.

The requirement to always promote the best interests of the patient would rule out all non-therapeutic studies involving risk. It would rule out phase I clinical trials (which look for any evidence of biological utility) which expose patients to risks with little hope of benefits, unless one construes interests to include long-term interests in finding a cure for their disease, or contributing to knowledge, or helping others, etc.[10]

The Declaration of Helsinki (paragraph 8) goes on to state:

> *'While the primary purpose of medical research is to generate new knowledge, this goal can never take precedence over the rights and interests of individual research subjects.'*[7]

A central ethical position taken by international and national guidelines is that research participants must be protected from being at much risk of harm, even if the benefit of the research to people in the future is considerable. There are two relevant components: the probability of the harm and the degree of harm. These are combined in the single term 'risk of harm', and the phrase 'minimal risk of harm' is often used to describe an acceptable level. Few guidelines specify what probability of serious harm (e.g., death) corresponds with 'minimal harm'. This nettle has been grasped by the Royal College of Physicians. A guideline in 1990 states that: '…Minimal risk could include everyday risks such as travelling on public transport or a private car … but would not include travel by pedal or motorcycle.'[14]

However, the guidance was later modified to join the Council of Europe in rejecting any risk of serious harm: 'the research bears minimal risk if it is to be expected that it would result, at the most, in a very slight and temporary negative impact on the health of the person concerned. We believe that this is the most acceptable definition in practice.'[15]

Two points are noteworthy about the position taken by these and other guidelines. First, they markedly restrict the degree of risk that competent adults can take voluntarily when participating in medical research. Even the 1990 definition was in marked contrast with many areas of life, such as sports. We allow people to cycle or ride motorbikes! Under the current definition, still more daily activities would be considered too risky if they were to come under the purview of research. Second, within the acceptable limits of risk, some tradeoff is allowed (in some guidelines) between risk to participants and the value of research to those in the future.

REASONABLE RISK VERSUS 'EQUIPOISE'

The gold standard of clinical research is the controlled clinical trial. This involves testing some new intervention either against placebo (or, if there is an existing intervention, against that intervention) as a 'trial'. To reduce bias, doctors are 'blinded' (when this is possible) so they do not know whether they are administering the experimental or control intervention.

It is commonly thought that randomised trials are only ethical if 'equipoise' exists. Equipoise is the idea that evidence does not favour either the new experimental intervention or the existing standard of care. That is, that professionals are genuinely uncertain which really is better. If professionals believe that one intervention is better, equipoise is disturbed and the trial must be stopped. This is in accordance with the eighth principle of the Declaration of Helsinki.[7]

However, these stringent ethical principles are virtually never met in randomised controlled trials. As we have noted, in order to justify clinical trials, clinicians must be uncertain whether some new treatment A is superior to existing treatment B. But there is almost always some evidence to suggest that A would be better (otherwise no one would bother doing the trial). As soon as any data accrue to shift confidence from 50/50, equipoise is disturbed. Imagine that, after 20 patients have been treated with a new cancer drug, 6 out of 10 patients treated with drug A have gone into remission, while only 4 patients out of ten treated with B have gone into remission. It looks like treatment A has a 60% chance of remission, while treatment B has only 40%. Beyond this point, trials continue in order to gain higher and higher levels of confidence that A is better than B. It may be that actually the initial results favoured drug A only by chance, or it may be that serious side effects from drug A would become apparent if the trial continued. Continuing the trial to involve more people protects future patients and ensures cost-effective use of limited resources. But as soon as there is some evidence that one treatment is better than the other, it is not in the trial participants' interests to continue – it exposes half the participants to risk of harm.[16] Equipoise is always disturbed in clinical research, well before trials are terminated.

Such decisions around equipoise have literally life and death implications for patients. To take just one example, in the classic Second International Study of Infarct Survival (ISIS-2) trial from the late 1980s, before the start of that trial, a large metaanalysis was performed which showed that thrombolytics ('clot busters' such as streptokinase) reduced the risk of death after heart attack by approximately 20% at the $P < 0.001$ level (odds ratio 0.78; 95% confidence interval (CI) 0.69 to 0.90).[17]

It is worth diverting at this point to describe so-called 'P values', for those who are not familiar with them. These numbers are a way of quantifying statistical uncertainty. They are a value between 0 and 1 that expresses the probability of observing by chance a particular result (or a more extreme one), given a certain statistical model. For example, in our example of the cancer drugs A and B, we could calculate a P value of 0.66.[a] This implies that there is a 66% chance, even if A and B are actually equally effective against the cancer, that out of 20 patients we would observe six remissions from drug A and four from drug B. This P value means that we wouldn't be terribly confident that drug A is better than B. They could be just as good, or B might be better. If we found the same pattern after studying 40 patients (12 remissions with drug A, 8 remissions with drug B), the P value would fall to 0.34. In 100 patients, the same pattern would have a 7% chance of occurring by chance ($P = 0.07$), while in 1000 patients (300 remissions with drug A, 200 remissions with drug B), the P value would be <0.0001, i.e., 0.01% probability of there appearing to be a difference occurring by chance and the drugs actually being equally effective. You can see that larger trials (with more patients in them) can generate more confidence in the results.

In scientific studies, a low P value (for example, arbitrarily defined as less than a value of 0.05) is sometimes regarded as 'statistically significant'. However, P values have to be interpreted. Just because something is statistically significant does not always mean that it is clinically significant. (In a large enough study, it might be possible to prove that a particular drug reduces the duration of your headache by 1 minute. But does that really matter?) Moreover, P values in themselves do not justify a particular scientific or policy conclusion.[18]

In the case of the streptokinase trials, the low P value from previous trials was not apparently regarded as conclusive, so the ISIS-2 trial[19] was commenced (despite another large Italian study

---

[a]Using Fisher's exact test.

being underway). Over the span of this study, there were 238 more deaths in the group receiving placebo compared with the group receiving streptokinase. This study found (unsurprisingly) that streptokinase reduced the risk of death by 23% (P <0.00001, 95% CI 18% to 32%).[20] US ethicist Baruch Brody puts the estimates of unnecessary deaths even higher, at around 400.[21]

Early in the trial, when only 4000 of around 17,000 patients had been randomised, the data monitoring committee stated that there was 'proof beyond reasonable doubt' that streptokinase worked. Why was the trial continued? It was to convince clinicians. As the chairman of the data monitoring committee, the legendary Sir Richard Doll (who discovered the link between smoking and lung cancer) put it: 'Involving large numbers of clinicians in the trial predisposes them to accept the results … Participation in a large-scale controlled trial constitutes, in practice, one of the best means of continuing medical education.'[22]

Such large trials are said to be necessary in practice to convince clinicians. But this justification is mistaken. The real issue is what level of confidence should change a clinician's mind. Sometimes practice ought to change. It may be true that clinicians will change their practice if the P value is <0.0001 but still, perhaps, we ought to stop trials earlier and change clinicians' minds in other ways – or even form binding policy. 'The question of what is the right "p value" to aim for, requires balancing the interests of trial participants, future patients and justice.'[23]

The Declaration of Helsinki attempts to address this difficult ethical issue by stating: 'When the risks are found to outweigh the potential benefits or when there is conclusive proof of definitive outcomes, physicians must assess whether to continue, modify or immediately stop the study.'[7]

But what constitutes 'conclusive'? The definition would be different for a parent of a dying baby, an administrator responsible for allocating resources or a treating clinician.

It is also an open and ethical question whether this is the best way to change practice. Perhaps we ought to be aggressively educating clinicians, or constructing mandatory best practice guidelines or informing patients of existing data, instead of subjecting half of the patients at risk of dying to placebo in a medical education exercise?

Elsewhere, one of us has discussed eight possible ways of making decisions about when there is 'enough evidence'.[20]

Strategy 1: Continue until certainty

One approach is to say that the trial should be continued until the 'right' answer is known. However, this is an illusion. Invariably, all we have is greater or lesser degrees of probability or confidence that the two treatments being compared differ in efficacy.

Strategy 2: Utilitarianism: maximise utility

According to this rule, the trial should be stopped at the point that would lead to the best outcome (e.g., fewest deaths) overall – taking both trial subjects and future patients whose treatment is affected by the trial into account and giving equal consideration to people in both groups.

This rule is likely to favour running trials until they are very large and the P values are very, very small – at least if the treatment of very large numbers of future patients is likely to be affected by the trial results. If we make a mistake and conclude that drug A is better than drug B when in fact B is better than A, a large number of people in the future will die through getting the worse treatment.

Strategy 3: Minimal evidence criterion

The central criticism for following the 'utilitarian' view is that it harms those in the trial for the sake of people in the future, thus conflicting with the Declaration of Helsinki.

As an alternative, a clinician should put the interests of his patients above all other concerns and pull out of the trial as soon as there is reasonable minimum evidence that one drug is better (for example, at a level statistical significance of P <0.05).

Strategy 4: When there is no longer 'reasonable uncertainty'

Strategies 2 and 3 assume no side effects. In practice though, drugs can have both short- and long-term unwanted effects. Because of this, different clinicians (and patients) might reasonably differ in their judgment as to when it is in their patients' best interests to receive treatment A or B, which would justify a clinician entering a patient into a trial on the grounds that there is reasonable uncertainty as to which is better overall, in the long term. This may be the case even if the minimal evidence condition is met with regard to the central outcome measure of the trial and justify running a trial for longer than would be the case using strategy 3.

Strategy 5: Clinical autonomy

We mentioned earlier the idea of equipoise in trials. According to the equipoise principle, patients can only be enrolled in a trial if the responsible doctor is genuinely uncertain which of the treatments would be best. Trials could continue until no doctors are willing to enrol their patients.

However, this strategy simply transfers the question of what the correct stopping rule is from the researcher to the clinician. More crucially, if individual clinicians are responsible for deciding whether it is right to enter a patient into a trial, they need to be provided with the latest data from the trial. But this is not generally done – partly to avoid the problem of bias, and also to prevent clinicians from losing equipoise. If clinicians are only given the evidence at the time before the start of the trial, they do not have available the data crucial to the question of whether the trial should be stopped.

Strategy 6: Pragmatism: what changes practice

Richard Doll gave two justifications for large clinical trials:
   1. They provide evidence that is 'much more readily accepted by clinicians'.
   2. 'Involving large numbers of clinicians in the trial predisposes them to accept the results.[24]
But this is putting the cart before the horse. We should first decide on what, epistemologically and ethically, are the correct criteria for stopping the trial, and then tackle the question of how clinicians' prescribing can be affected. It is wrong to continue trials beyond reasonable evidence and expose participants to inferior treatment simply as a means of correcting clinicians' poor prescribing habits.

Strategy 7: When potential subjects are better off outside the trial

The pragmatic argument could be applied more convincingly in considering only the best interests of those in the trial. Different clinicians make different judgments about when to switch to a new treatment. Such differences might be reasonable, given uncertainties over the longer-term side effects of the new treatment. According to strategy 7, when the interim analysis shows (with conventional levels of significance, such as $P < 0.05$) that treatment A is better than treatment B, the trial leaders should ask the following question to the clinicians involved: 'Given this information, if the trial were stopped now, which treatment would you recommend for your patients?' If the clinician answered B – but was still willing to randomise – then it would be best to continue the trial, recruiting patients from this clinician. If the clinician answered A, then it would be best to discontinue the trial, even if the clinician were willing to randomise.

Strategy 8: The autonomy of patients

All the strategies so far have concentrated on the question of when those running the trial, or clinicians, should stop it. The interests of the patients taking part in the trial have been considered but not their views. Yet, if we are concerned about ethics, surely patients should be involved in the decision concerning their entry into the trial? Almost always, a minimum standard should be that patients are informed about the trial and the fact that it is a randomised controlled trial. But they are rarely given emerging evidence from a trial. One response to the problem of when to terminate trials is to allow participants to access emerging data and decide whether to participate.

Where there is scientific and medical controversy relating to research, one of us (DW) has suggested a version of the Patient Autonomy approach of informing participants, or their parents, of professional uncertainty. He calls this the Equal Airtime approach:

During elections, one way of improving voters' ability to make informed decisions is to provide legitimate political parties with equal opportunities to present their point of view. A similar strategy in the setting of the debate about controlled trials would be to provide research participants with the case for and against participation in a trial. This could take the form of a two-page information summary, with the evidence and arguments in favour of participation in a trial on one side of a page and the corresponding evidence against participation presented on the other. The equal airtime alternative could be invoked where a particular threshold has been reached; for example, where there is evidence of statistically significant net benefit or harm from an adequately powered previous trial or metaanalysis, and where there is reasonable disagreement about whether or not a trial should take place. The researchers would provide the case for participation, while those clinicians or researchers who feel that controlled trials should not continue could provide the case against a trial.[25]

'NOTHING TO LOSE': CHOOSING PARTICIPANTS WITH THE LEAST TO LOSE

We have looked at whether trials should start, and when or if they should stop. But who should be enrolled in trials? The healthy or the sick? What about the sickest of patients, or those with the worst forms of an illness? They often aren't eligible to be involved in trials – perhaps because they are not able to consent, because they might be more sensitive to side effects or because they are regarded as vulnerable to coercion.

The case of Jesse Gelsinger is particularly relevant. In 1999, Jesse was an 18-year-old man with a mild form of a rare genetic metabolic disorder – ornithine transcarbamylase (OTC) deficiency. Jesse's form of the disease could be controlled by diet and drug treatment. A more severe form of the disease occurs in newborns and is often lethal or requires infants to have a liver transplant. Researchers had been working on a new gene therapy for OTC deficiency. Gelsinger was recruited into a trial of gene therapy: he was injected with virus vector particles containing a gene to correct the genetic defect. However, tragically, Gelsinger developed a massive immune response to the virus and became gravely ill with multiorgan failure. He died 4 days later. This was the first death directly attributed to gene therapy.[26]

In designing the trial, the researchers had decided, on ethical advice, to recruit adult participants who could consent but who had a mild form of the disease, rather than newborns who could not consent but had a lethal form of the disease.[26] Consent was considered more important than minimising expected harm.

This case illustrates the importance of distinguishing between two concepts: the chances of a bad outcome occurring and expected harm. The magnitude of the expected harm to adult participants with milder forms of this disease was significantly greater than to newborns with the severe form of the disease. Gelsinger had something to lose (his whole life of near normal quality), while a seriously affected newborn did not (he or she stood to lose months of poor quality life).

In another court case, the judge noted:

> 'Where there is no alternative treatment available and the disease is progressive and fatal, it seems to me to be reasonable to consider experimental treatment with unknown benefits and risks, but without significant risks of increased suffering to the patient, in cases where there is some chance of benefit to the patient. A patient who is not able to consent to pioneering treatment ought not to be deprived of the chance in circumstances where he would have been likely to consent if he had been competent.'[27]

This has important implications for newborn babies like Charlie Gard. Such infants potentially have little to lose from taking part in research.

A principle of minimising expected harm implies that research should be conducted on newborns with the poorest prognosis. For any given risk, the lower the expected harm is, the worse the prognosis of the infant.

REASONABLE RISK

In considering whether or not to allow experimental treatment, we cannot rely on a statistically arbitrary threshold, nor on a vague concept like that of 'minimal harm'. There may be reasonable disagreement about where we should draw the bar for each of these. Perhaps, instead, we could draw on the concept of reasonableness?

In determining whether the risks of participation in research are reasonable, the following factors are relevant[28]:

1. Is there a known risk to participants prior to commencing the study, and what is its magnitude, based on evidence available at the time?
2. Should any nonhuman or epidemiological research, systematic overview or computer modelling have been performed prior to the study to better estimate the risk to participants or obviate the need for the use of human participants?
3. Could the risk have been reduced in any other way? Is it as small as possible?
4. Are the potential benefits (in terms of knowledge or improvement of welfare of trial participants or other people) of this study worth the risks?
5. Could this research generate knowledge that is likely to significantly harm either participants or others outside the research, now or in the future?

Many people have a black and white view of medical ethics. They believe some course of action is right or wrong, or some treatment is proven or unproven. But in many cases, there is not only black and white, but also grey. Sometimes we are in the grey zone of ethics, where it is not possible to say which of two options is better. The options may differ in the probabilities of their outcomes (or confidence in the quality of the evidence), or in length or quality of life on offer.

A very prominent example of the reasonableness of more than one option is the case of Ashya King.

In 2014, Ashya King was a 5-year-old boy who had been diagnosed with a form of malignant brain tumour called medulloblastoma. Ashya received surgery to remove the tumour at Southampton General Hospital in July 2014, which appeared to be a success.[29] Follow-up treatment of chemotherapy and radiotherapy was required, since medulloblastoma can spread in the brain and spinal cord and has a high rate of recurring if treated with surgery alone.

There are two types of radiotherapy. Photon (or x-ray–based) radiotherapy is the traditional kind of radiotherapy and was offered by the NHS at the time. It involves exposing the whole brain and spinal cord to radiation to try to kill any remaining tumour cells. However, this treatment can have serious long-term side effects, including problems with growth, hormone production, additional cancers and learning.

Ashya King's parents had read on the internet about a new form of radiotherapy, proton therapy, which promised similar results but with fewer side effects in some cancers. It was not available at that time in the UK, but it was available abroad. At that time, the NHS would pay for patients to have proton therapy abroad. Concerned about side effects, Ashya's parents declined consent for the standard treatment and asked for him to receive this new treatment instead. Following this request, Ashya's consultant applied for funding to allow him to access treatment in Prague. Specialists at a proton therapy centre there had treated other children with medulloblastoma and were willing to treat Ashya. However, the NHS funding panel declined the request. Funding was not extended to patients with medulloblastoma tumours, on the basis that it was not clear that proton therapy would actually result in fewer side effects, and because of concern that logistical delays (due to travel and starting treatment) might worsen the outcome of treatment.[30]

Following a breakdown in communication with the medical team, Ashya's parents claimed that they were told that if they sought the treatment themselves, the hospital would seek an emergency protection order to prevent it. (In a later court hearing, the hospital denied this, saying that 'the Trust had never opposed the family's decision to obtain proton therapy. The Trust itself was not in a position to offer it, but would support it being provided elsewhere if it could be reliably arranged and funded and the transfer arrangements were safe.'[30])

On August 28th, his parents took Ashya from the hospital and transported him to France, and then to Spain, where they had property. They planned to obtain funds for his treatment in Prague. On August 29th, the hospital filed an application to make Ashya a ward of court and to direct his medical treatment. This was awarded, and Ashya was taken to hospital in Malaga, without having suffered any apparent harm from the travel. Ashya's parents were arrested using a European Arrest Warrant.[31]

The case of Ashya King was heard, urgently, by the High Court. At the first hearing, on September 2nd, the Crown Prosecution Service indicated to court that they would drop the European Arrest Warrant. The hospital also indicated it did not oppose the proton therapy treatment, although it could not fund it. The case was adjourned until the parents could be present. During telephone hearings over the next 2 days, the court ordered Ashya's parents to detail the nature of the treatment planned and asked the hospital to respond. On September 5th, the court received confirmation that the Prague Hospital had a treatment plan in place, that transport was in place and that funds were in place for the transport and treatment. Justice Baker therefore ordered that the plan to travel to Prague could go ahead. On September 8th, Ashya was admitted to hospital in Prague. This was 6 weeks and 4 days after the operation.

In this case, the question was not what was 'best practice' for Ashya, or what was usual care. It was whether the option the parents wanted to choose was reasonable, even if the alternative course was also reasonable. The court considered Aysha's welfare and his right to life and to a family life. It stated that the court should only intervene if the child was at risk of being harmed by the parents failing to reach a reasonable standard of parental care.

The judge summarised very succinctly the importance of imprecision in ethics:

'In some cases, this court is faced with a dispute between medical authorities and parents who are insisting on a wholly unreasonable course of treatment, or withholding consent to an essential therapy for their child – for example, a blood transfusion. This is manifestly not such a case. The course of treatment proposed by Mr and Mrs King is entirely reasonable. Ashya has a serious medical condition. Any parents in the position of Mr and Mrs King would do whatever they could to explore all options. Some parents would follow the advice of the local doctors to use conventional radiotherapy, others would prefer the relatively untested option of proton therapy (assuming the funds can be made available to meet the cost of transport and treatment) in the hope that the toxic effects of radiation will be reduced. Both courses are reasonable and it is the parents who bear

the heavy responsibility of making the decision. It is no business of this court, or any other public authority, to interfere with their decision.'[30]

When new options are tried, it is important that these are treated in a scientific way. It is important that scientific appraisal is done wherever possible, and more evidence is accumulated, so that we can see which option is really better. Thus, when two options are reasonable, it is important to continue to audit their effects. In an age where massive amounts of data can be collected and manipulated ('Big Data'), there is a moral imperative to measure all interventions as systematically as possible.

In 2016, a nonrandomised phase II study published in the Lancet showed that proton therapy had similar outcomes and fewer side effects to photon therapy.[32]

From 2017, proton beam therapy became available with in the UK.

EXPERT EVIDENCE AND THE STANDARD OF CARE

We discussed whether there was enough evidence in support of treatment. But a different question is whether there are enough experts in favour? In Ashya's case, there were some specialists who were in favour of the new form of radiotherapy. In an earlier case, very similar to that of Charlie Gard, there was debate about whether there was enough support.[28]

In 2002, the High Court heard another case of two adolescents with an advanced stage of Creutzfeldt Jakob disease (CJD). An 18-year-old Jonathan Simms and a 16-year-old girl (known as 'A') both had this rare neurodegenerative disease and had become severely disabled, with the prospect of dying within a short period. There was no cure for their condition and no available treatment able to either prolong their lives or stop their neurological decline.

In a parallel with the Gard case, some preliminary scientific evidence suggested a treatment that reduced the formation of the toxic prion protein in mice with a different form of the disease. However, there was a catch. The treatment (pentosan polysulphate) had never been tested in humans and also required surgery so that treatment could be given directly into the fluid spaces in the brain.

Jonathan Simms' and A's parents sought a court declaration allowing their children to have the treatment. They believed that their children would have wanted to try this treatment.

In UK negligence law, one of the standards of the duty of care a doctor owes his or her patient is known as the Bolam test:

> *'the standard of the ordinary skilled man exercising and professing to have that special skill. A man need not possess the highest expert skill at the risk of being found negligent. It is a well-established law that it is sufficient if he exercises the ordinary skill of an ordinary man exercising that particular art.'*[33]

According to the Bolam test, a doctor would not be found negligent if they had acted in accordance with the practice of 'a responsible body' of medical opinion – i.e., if a good number of his or her peers would have acted similarly.

In the court case of experimental treatment for CJD, there was no question of negligence. Nevertheless, the court asked whether there was a responsible body of medical opinion within the United Kingdom who would support the experimental treatment. The judge, Dame Butler-Sloss, said the answer was unclear.[28] The treatment was untried in humans and there was no validation of the experimental work done in Japan. However, the judge went further and argued that this was the wrong standard to apply.

'The "Bolam test" ought not to be allowed to inhibit medical progress. And it is clear that if one waited for the "Bolam test" to be complied with to its fullest extent, no innovative work such as the use of penicillin or performing heart transplant surgery would ever be attempted.'[28]

The court heard contrasting opinions from medical experts. A Japanese neuropathologist who had studied the drug in animal experiments supported the treatment. A neurosurgeon who had been approached by the families was prepared to support the families' request for treatment and perform the surgical procedure. Two consultant neurologists gave evidence: one cautiously supported the families, while the other was more pessimistic about the treatment and did not believe that it was in Jonathan's or A's interests to receive pentosan.

How should we decide which expert to believe? We will return to the question of expert disagreement in Chapter 7, but here we will note the insights of the political philosopher John Rawls.

Rawls described a process to develop the principles of justice that he called 'reflective equilibrium'. This involves first developing general principles and concepts, but then, crucially, revising these in line with intuitions about specific cases. This process is what judges engage in when they make decisions; but judges, or doctors, are not necessarily or exclusively ethical experts.

Rawls described the qualities of people who should be engaged in reflective equilibrium. He calls them 'competent judges'. They should be knowledgeable about the facts and of the consequences of the various courses of action. Importantly, they should be 'reasonable'. There are four criteria for reasonableness: (1) being willing to use inductive logic, (2) being disposed to find reasons for and against a solution, (3) having an open mind and (4) making a conscientious effort to overcome one's intellectual, emotional and moral prejudices.[34] Lastly, a reasonable person is to have 'sympathetic knowledge … of those human interests which, by conflicting in particular cases, give rise to the need to make a moral decision.'

In the case of Jonathan Simms and A, Justice Butler-Sloss felt that those supporting treatment were reasonable, and that there was enough expert support. She decided in favour of providing the experimental treatment, and subsequently both patients received pentosan. (While Jonathan Simms survived for much longer than expected, more recent published scientific reports of the treatment from UK and Japan do not appear to show any overall neurological improvements in patients with CJD.[b])

The cases of Jonathan Simms and A appear remarkably similar to Charlie Gard's case. Why was a different decision reached in this case?

One major difference was that these were adolescents, not babies, and their parents claimed they would have wanted a trial of therapy. We will return in the next chapter to the difference between adults (or young adults) and infants, but it would potentially be reasonable to take greater risks in embarking on experimental treatment where the patient understands and is willing to take on those risks (or at least there is good reason to think that they would have been).

A second major difference is the degree of brain damage at the time of the court case, as well as dependence on intensive forms of medical life support.

In Charlie's case, he was paralysed, apparently unable to respond to his environment and on a breathing machine in intensive care. Both his parents and health professionals agreed that his current life was not worth prolonging.

---

[b]A review article in 2013 concluded: 'Albeit promising, findings to date fail to illustrate any reversal of clinical manifestations or recovery of pre-existing neurological deficits in patients.' Some patients appeared to show prolonged survival.[35]

Jonathan and A were also severely disabled. However, they were both reported to be able to recognise their family and respond to them. For example, Jonathan was described as very affectionate, and kissed his family. He responded to music (indicating which music he liked). He apparently watched soccer on television with his father and was excited when his team scored.

The judge noted:

> 'No-one who knows them or has seen them, whether the consultants who gave evidence, the members of both families, other doctors or nurses, have suggested that either JS or JA has no quality of life, nor that they cannot respond to their parents and others, nor that they cannot feel pleasure and pain ... I am satisfied that both JS and JA have the ability, even now at a late stage of this disease, to feel pleasure and pain and have some enjoyment from life which is worth preserving.'[28]

ALL ADVANCES START FROM SOMEWHERE

In Ashya's case, there was some evidence and some experience with proton therapy in medulloblastoma. In the case of the patients with CJD, there was some scientific evidence, but the treatment had not been tested on humans.

However, it is important to remember that many advances have been made (including the first antileukaemia drugs) through experimental trial and error.

Dr Sidney Farber, the famous pathologist whose memory is now acknowledged by the successful, international Dana-Farber Cancer Institute, has long been heralded as providing the first successful cure for childhood acute lymphoblastic leukaemia (ALL). What is sometimes forgotten in this case is that Dr Farber initially used experimental therapy. Building on an observation from a doctor treating anaemia with folic acid, he presumed folic acid might be a good therapy for ALL. His first treatment actually caused acceleration of disease, and multiple patients died quickly from uncontrolled leukaemia. However, this observation lead Dr Farber to try the reverse, an antifolic acid medication. Again, in an experimental, non–evidence-based practice, he trialled his new therapy. The result was the beginning of a cure for ALL and medications that are still the mainstay of therapy today.

The judicial system relies heavily upon the expert medical opinion, which in turn is based upon evidence-based practice. In the case of Charlie Gard, the treatment in the US that the parents were seeking was deemed experimental therapy with a low chance of providing benefit or cure. However, this is not absolute. As exemplified by the case of ALL, experimental therapy, in rare cases, can provide the advances that one day underpin curative therapy.[c]

There are of course limits to aggressively offering experimental treatment:

1. Side effects of treatment may make it highly likely not to be in the individual's interests.
2. It is expensive, and (as discussed in the previous chapter) would deny other patients their slice of the limited health care pie.

However, if a treatment has never been tried, it may be impossible to know if there would be side effects or benefits – any assessment of best interests (as discussed in Chapter 3) would be impossible.

One alternative, in at least some cases, would be to provide a limited trial of therapy – to see whether any positive or negative effects arise. Where there is contention about an experimental treatment that is requested by a dying or severely ill patient (or their representative), perhaps it should be provided with a plan for active withdrawal? We will return to explore in more detail this possibility of time-limited trials of treatment in Chapter 8.

---

[c]Thanks to Rachel Conyers for these points.

Conclusion

Our aim in this chapter has been to identify and explore some of the value-based questions that apply to scientific research and innovative or experimental treatments. While science and scientific knowledge aspire to be objective, performing science and using that knowledge involves values. As a consequence, there will inevitably be different views about how to evaluate evidence and when to allow experimental treatment.

Even if the benefits of the research are only for other people in the future, that might be a benefit worth pursuing (for the child or for the parents) if the harm of research is small or nonexistent. That raises the problem of working out what the harm would be, as well as how much harm is minimal. The notion of clinician equipoise is valuable in randomised trials, yet this state of completely balanced evidence between two treatments is easily disrupted. The vital question of how long to continue trials when there is some evidence in favour of one treatment over another reflects the need to weigh up the interests of current versus future patients. For treatments that are in much earlier stages of development (for example, that have not yet been tried in humans), there can be understandable reluctance to try them out, particularly in patients who are very unwell. However, all innovations have to start from somewhere. These patients may also have the least to lose from participating in trials of novel therapy. We should not expect that cutting-edge treatments will be endorsed by the majority of experts or practicing doctors – these interventions will always be on the margins of current practice. We need some way of evaluating the credibility and reasonableness of those who are proposing the treatment.

Those questions may often be simpler in adults, since we can defer to the views of the patient. We can ensure that they understand the benefits and risks of taking part in the research and still wish to take part. We cannot do that for young children, but we can ask their parents. Why isn't that the answer? That is where we will turn next.

References

1. *Abrams v United States 250 U.S. 616* (1919).
2. *Great Ormond Street Hospital v Yates & Ors [2017] EWHC 972 (Fam) (11 April 2017) para 81.*
3. Hume, D. & Mossner, E. C. (1984) *A treatise of human nature.* London, Penguin Books. 3.1.1
4. Savulescu, J. (2000) The ethics of cloning and creating embryonic stem cells as a source of tissue for transplantation: time to change the law in Australia. *Aust N Z J Med,* 30, 492-8.
5. Savulescu, J., Chalmers, I. & Blunt, J. (1996) Are research ethics committees behaving unethically? Some suggestions for improving performance and accountability. *BMJ,* 313, 1390-3.
6. Kahneman, D. (2011). *Thinking, fast and slow.* New York: Farrar, Straus and Giroux.
7. World Medical Association. (2013). *'Declaration of Helsinki: ethical principles for medical research involving human subjects.'* Accessed 04/12/2008 from <https://www.wma.net/policies-post/wma-declaration-of-helsinki-ethical-principles-for-medical-research-involving-human-subjects/>.
8. (2005) *Mental Capacity Act.* Accessed from <https://www.legislation.gov.uk/ukpga/2005/9/contents>.
9. Savulescu, J. & Spriggs, M. (2002) The hexamethonium asthma study and the death of a normal volunteer in research. *J Med Ethics,* 28, 3-4.
10. Savulescu, J. (2017) The structure of ethics review: expert ethics committees and the challenge of voluntary research euthanasia. *J Med Ethics.* Published Online First: 07 September 2017. doi: 10.1136/medethics-2015-103183.
11. Brierley, J. & Shaw, D. (2016) Premortem interventions in dying children to optimise organ donation: an ethical analysis. *J Med Ethics,* 42, 424-8.
12. World Medical Association. (2017). *'Declaration of Geneva.'* From <https://www.wma.net/policies-post/wma-declaration-of-geneva/>.
13. World Medical Association. (2006). *'International Code of Medical Ethics.'* From <https://www.wma.net/policies-post/wma-international-code-of-medical-ethics/>.
14. Royal College of Physicians (1990) *Guidelines on the practice of ethics committees in medical research with human participants.* 2nd Edition. London.

15. Royal College of Physicians (2007) *Guidelines on the practice of ethics committees in medical research with human participants.* 4th Edition ed. Accessed from <https://shop.rcplondon.ac.uk/products/guidelines-on-the-practice-of-ethics-committees-in-medical-research-with-human-participants?variant=6364998469>.

16. Savulescu, J. & Hope, T. (2010) Ethics of Research. in J. Skorupski (Ed.) *The Routledge companion to ethics.* Abingdon, Routledge, pp. 781-95.

17. Yusuf, S., Collins, R., Peto, R., Furberg, C., Stampfer, M. J., Goldhaber, S. Z., et al. (1985) Intravenous and intracoronary fibrinolytic therapy in acute myocardial infarction: overview of results on mortality, reinfarction and side-effects from 33 randomized controlled trials. *Eur Heart J,* 6, 556-85.

18. Wasserstein, R. & Lazar, N. (2016) The ASA's statement on p-values: context, process, and purpose. *The American Statistician,* 70, 129-133.

19. (1988) Randomised trial of intravenous streptokinase, oral aspirin, both, or neither among 17,187 cases of suspected acute myocardial infarction: ISIS-2. ISIS-2 (Second International Study of Infarct Survival) Collaborative Group. *Lancet,* 2, 349-60.

20. Savulescu, J. & Hope, T. (2010) Ethics of Research. in J. Skorupski (Ed.) *The Routledge companion to ethics.* Abingdon, Routledge, pp. 781-95.

21. Brody, B. A. (1995) *Ethical issues in drug testing, approval, and pricing : the clot-dissolving drugs.* New York; Oxford, Oxford University Press.

22. Doll, R. (1993) Summation of the Conference. Doing more good than harm: the evaluation of health care interventions. *Ann N Y Acad Sci,* 703, 310-13.

23. Savulescu, J. (2015) Bioethics: why philosophy is essential for progress. *J Med Ethics,* 41, 28-33.

24. Doll, R. (1993) Summation of the Conference. Doing more good than harm: the evaluation of health care interventions. *Ann N Y Acad Sci,* 703, 310-13.

25. Wilkinson, D. (2010) Therapeutic hypothermia and the 'equal air-time' solution for controversial randomised trials. *J Paediatr Child Health,* 46, 577-8.

26. Savulescu, J. (2001) Harm, ethics committees and the gene therapy death. *J Med Ethics,* 27, 148-50.

27. *Simms v An NHS Trust [2002] EWHC 2734 (Fam) (11 December 2002) para 57.*

28. Savulescu, J. (1998b) Commentary: safety of participants in non-therapeutic research must be ensured. *BMJ,* 316, 891-2; discussion 893-4.

29. Bridgeman, J. (2015) Misunderstanding, threats, and fear, of the law in conflicts over children's healthcare: in the matter of Ashya King [2014] EWHC 2964. *Med Law Rev,* 23, 477-89.

30. *In the matter of Ashya King (A child) [2014] EWHC 2964.*

31. O'Brien, A. & Sokol, D. K. (2014) Lessons from the Ashya King case. *BMJ,* 349, g5563.

32. Yock, T. I., Yeap, B. Y., Ebb, D. H., Weyman, E., Eaton, B. R., Sherry, N. A., et al. (2016) Long-term toxic effects of proton radiotherapy for paediatric medulloblastoma: a phase 2 single-arm study. *Lancet Oncol,* 17, 287-98.

33. *Bolam v Friern Hospital Management committee [1957] 1 WLR 583.*

34. Rawls, J. (1951) Outline of a decision procedure for ethics. *Philosophical Review,* 60, 177-97.

35. Panegyres, P. K. & Armari, E. (2013) Therapies for human prion diseases. *Am J Neurodegener Dis,* 2, 176-86.

CHAPTER 6

Parents

'*Children begin by loving their parents; after a time they judge them; rarely, if ever, do they forgive them.*'
Oscar Wilde

'*And is not that a Mother's gentle hand that undraws your curtains, and a Mother's sweet voice that summons you to rise? To rise and forget, in the bright sunlight, the ugly dreams that frightened you so when all was dark.*'
An Easter Greeting to Every Child Who Loves Alice, Lewis Carroll

'*Some people may ask why the court has any function in this process, why can the parents not just make the decision for themselves?*'[1]
JUSTICE FRANCIS, APRIL 11

'*the decisive issue is whether the fair balance that must exist between the competing interests at stake – those of the child, of the two parents, and of public order – has been struck, within the margin of appreciation afforded to States in such matters, taking into account, however, that the best interests of the child must be of primary consideration.*'[2]
EUROPEAN COURT OF HUMAN RIGHTS, JUNE 20

In previous chapters, we have discussed some of the difficulties in determining what the right course of action would have been for Charlie – or in other cases of disputed treatment. Given these difficulties many observers had asked themselves the question highlighted by Justice Francis. Why, ultimately, isn't it the parents' decision to make?

To understand this, it is important to appreciate the difference between decisions about medical treatment for children and decisions for adults. Imagine an adult equivalent of the Charlie Gard case:

Colin Giles is a young adult with a severe, progressive and incurable brain disorder. He is now unconscious and dependent on life support in intensive care. Doctors believe that his outlook is extremely poor and continuing treatment would be 'futile'. Before Colin became more unwell, though, he had been actively researching possible treatments for his condition. He had told his partner Carla that he did not want her to give up hope. In particular, Colin wanted to receive a trial of an experimental treatment that was under development, but hadn't yet been tested. Colin told Carla that if he deteriorated and was on life support in intensive care, he would not want doctors to stop life support. He would want life support to be continued so that he could have a trial of the experimental treatment. Colin knew that there was little chance that this treatment would work, and understood that intensive care might be unpleasant – but he still wished such a trial to go ahead. Carla has successfully raised funds for Colin to travel overseas for treatment. Should this be allowed?

In a case like that of Colin Giles, there would be a major focus on his views when competent about treatment.[a] Why? An adult's wishes might conflict with what would actually be best for him. In some situations, the patient's views might be idiosyncratic, based on religion or other supernatural beliefs, or unreasonable. (Imagine that Colin's decision to choose this particular experimental treatment was because he liked the name of the drug, or because he had seen a picture of the doctor offering the treatment and thought that she looked attractive.) Perhaps we feel that Colin has made an unwise choice, and that it would be much better to accept his mortality and not prolong his dying in intensive care. He should, you might believe, die with dignity. Nevertheless, as long as Colin had capacity at the time that he indicated his wishes, the usual principle is that doctors should try to respect his previous wishes. So, in this imagined case, if there is good evidence that the adult Colin had wanted to be kept alive on a ventilator, if he would have wanted to pursue experimental treatment overseas, despite the apparently slim chance of benefit (and, from our discussion in Chapter 4, as long as this would be within the boundaries of distributive justice and consistent with fair allocation of limited healthcare resources), there is a strong argument that treatment should be provided or continued. It seems far less likely that the hypothetical case of Colin Giles would reach the court, and if it had reached the court, it seems more likely that the decision would have ultimately been in favour of providing treatment.

The ethical difference between the hypothetical Colin Giles and the real Charlie Gard case is in two separate ways. First, when thinking about decisions in medical ethics for adults, we give significant weight to patient autonomy. Autonomy refers to the value of self-determination, or a right to make decisions about one's own life. For medicine, it is about respecting patients' wishes about medical treatment. Autonomy is often understood as freedom from interference – it is a negative right. Because of that, there is a very strong belief that patients' refusal of treatment must be respected. We would allow an adult to refuse a blood transfusion or to decline cancer treatment, even if those treatments would be life-saving and with few side effects.

There is less significance of autonomy in patient requests for treatment.[3] Autonomy does not mean that patients have a positive right to whatever treatment they choose. However, even if we don't think that autonomy gives patients a right to demand treatment, nevertheless, respecting patient autonomy gives us a separate (and potentially strong) reason to provide treatment if the patient desires it and there are no other good reasons against doing so.

Second, if we are trying to determine what would be in a patient's best interests, their values and wishes are important. It is difficult to know how to weigh up the risks and benefits of experimental treatment. But a previously expressed desire for this treatment (despite uncertainties and risks) would be relevant to determining what would be best for Colin Giles. While this obviously overlaps with the argument based on autonomy, there is a more nuanced relationship between someone's wishes and best interests. If Colin's desire for treatment is part of longstanding values that were important to him, that gives us extra reason to think that treatment would be in his own best interests. (If his expressed desire had been more transient, or less obviously related to values that were central to him, we might feel that this was less relevant to his interests.)

For example, a person might request that mechanical ventilation be continued because he believes that we should not intervene in God's will. Such beliefs are arguably irrational,

[a]'Competence' here is a term that refers to people's ability to make decisions. A competent patient is one who is able understand, recall and weigh up the important factors relevant to a decision.

even in religious terms.[4] However, they are frequently respected. It is also important not to discriminate against secular nonreligious beliefs. If a person requests ongoing ventilation because she does not believe in an afterlife and believes that the Singularity is coming and she will be able to upload into an artificial intelligence, that belief ought to be accorded the same respect.[5]

In the real Charlie Gard case, however, we could not give any weight to the autonomy of the patient, to Charlie's wishes. He was never in a position to understand his medical condition or to develop values relevant to the decision. His parents, though, clearly did have values and views about his treatment.

What significance should be placed on the autonomy or the wishes of parents in cases of disputed treatment for children?

Parental autonomy

One view might be that parental autonomy is just like autonomy for adult patients. We allow patients to make decisions about medical treatment because it is their life and their body. As long as they aren't harming anyone else, why should it be anyone else's business whether they decide to have a particular medical treatment? Some might suggest that parents have a right to decide about treatment because it is their child and their family.

But the autonomy of parents is very obviously different from the autonomy of patients to make decisions for themselves. While adult patients are generally thought to have an absolute right to refuse medical treatment for themselves, we don't usually think that parents can refuse all medical treatment for their children.

As an example, in February 2017, a couple in Michigan refused medical treatment for their jaundiced newborn baby, Abigail. A midwife had visited and told the parents that the baby needed urgent treatment. However, Abigail's parents believed that she would be healed by prayer. The baby died 2 days later from complications of newborn jaundice (a medical condition that is readily treatable).[6] In cases like this, we don't think that parental autonomy gives parents a right to refuse treatment. There have to be some limits.

> 'Where, as in this case, the parents spend a great deal of time with their child, their views may have particular value because they know the patient and how he reacts so well … Their own wishes, however understandable in human terms, are wholly irrelevant to consideration of the objective best interests of the child save to the extent in any given case that they may illuminate the quality and value to the child of the child/parent relationship.'[7]

In the case of MB, an infant with severe muscular weakness (spinal muscular atrophy), the judge saw value in the parents' perspective on treatment. However, he distinguished between the views of parents and the wishes of parents. Is there reason to distinguish between parents' views and wishes in this way? How are they relevant to the child's best interests?

Knowledge of child

One reason to take parents' views into account is because of their knowledge of the child. If parents refuse antibiotics because they know that their child has previously had a serious allergic reaction to those same antibiotics, it would be vital to pay attention to their concerns. In an older child, parents will often be able to provide evidence about the day-to-day life of the child, what they like or dislike and how much their life is affected by illness or impairment. In Chapter 3, we discussed the significance for decisions of the burdens of treatment or illness, as well as the objective benefits of life-prolonging treatment. The views of parents may be highly relevant to an understanding of what life is really like for the child and hence whether it would be best to keep them alive or to allow them to die. However, sometimes parents' assessment may differ from that of others caring for the child, and it may not be clear whether parents' views are overly positive (because of an understandable strong desire that their child is improving), or whether professionals are overly negative. In the Gard case, Charlie's parents had spent hours at his bedside. They believed that he was aware of his surroundings and responding to them. In contrast, the nurses and doctors caring for Charlie in intensive care felt that he did not respond. A judgment may need to be made about which evidence should be believed. In the Gard case, the judge appeared to be more persuaded by the medical evidence.

Effect on child

Parents' views might, at least in some circumstances, influence whether or not treatment would be in a child's best interests. In Chapter 3, we mentioned the case of Y, an 8-year-old girl who had a longstanding spinal muscular atrophy. In that case, the judge indicated the importance for Y's quality of life of her family's care and devotion. She had 'a loving and supportive family who were acutely concerned with her wellbeing and are diligent in seeking to ensure that everything that can be done for her is done'. One of the medical consultants praised the 'care, love, devotion and expertise which Y's family lavished on her in supporting her through these technically demanding treatments for many years. Without their loving care and attention, Y would undoubtedly have died many years ago.'[8]

However, even with the most devoted parents in the world, there are limits to how much parents are able to influence the wellbeing of a child. Where a child's condition causes them to suffer or prevents them from appreciating or enjoying benefits from continuing life, the scales may still be tipped against treatment.

The judge in MB's case dismissed the 'wishes' of parents (as 'wholly irrelevant'), but that might be too hasty. There are two reasons to perhaps take these into account.

UNCERTAINTY

We have described in the previous chapters some of the challenges in determining whether treatment would work, how likely it is that it would work and how to weigh up the risks and benefits of treatment. In many situations, it isn't clear that there is a single right answer. There may be different reasonable views about whether to continue life support or discontinue life support, whether to provide experimental treatment or not.

Where there is genuine moral uncertainty (uncertainty about what is the right thing to do), we should, in general, allow parents to make decisions about treatment for a child. Why? Here, perhaps, is where parental autonomy and parental wishes are relevant – parents have a right to decide, within reasonable bounds, how to raise and care for their children. After the child, they will be the ones who are likely to be most affected by the decision. That especially includes decisions where there might be a range of different views about what to do. It would exclude situations that are clear-cut. In the case of the jaundiced baby Abigail, there is not any real uncertainty about what the right thing would have been. There is not likely to be reasonable disagreement about what her parents should have done. They should have taken her to a doctor.

In others cases, there is more uncertainty. Whether we prefer one course of action or another will depend on our values. Sometimes, faced with disagreement, the temptation may be to stay with the status quo – for example, to continue current treatment, or not to embark upon a requested procedure/treatment. However, that 'nondecision' is still a decision. It still involves a value judgment (about the current situation versus an alternative). We are morally responsible for the outcome because we could have acted otherwise. If there is real uncertainty about the right course (and as long as parents appear to be competent to decide), it would be unfair for courts or doctors to impose their own values on a family.

INTERESTS OF PARENTS AND OTHER FAMILY MEMBERS

Finally, one overlapping reason for allowing parents to make a decision (where there is uncertainty) is because these decisions have profound effects on the parents themselves and other members of the family. Where a decision would lead to a child surviving, that will often result in a substantial burden of care for other family members. Where the decision would lead to the child dying, in most cases it is the parents and family who will carry the greatest emotional burden of the loss of the child. It is they who will have to live with the decision.

Stepping outside of the intensive care unit and the hospital, if we think about other serious decisions that parents make for their children, it is usual for parents to take into account their own interests, as well as those of other members of the family. Every day, parents make decisions that affect the interests of their children. They decide what sort of food to provide, how to travel, how fast to drive, which school to send their children to, which activities to involve them in, whether to move house, which job to apply for. All of those decisions involve tradeoffs. It would be possible for parents who have a single child to make every decision based only on what (they feel) would be best for their child. However, it isn't clear that this is what we should expect of parents. Some might think that a perfect parent would pay attention to what would be best for their child and be prepared to make sacrifices for their child. However, it isn't even clear that that is the ideal for parenthood. Surely, we wouldn't expect parents to sacrifice all of their own interests and wellbeing as soon as they have a child? In any case, for parents with more than one child, that supposed ideal becomes impossible. Decisions that are the best for one child become less than the best for other children. Parents should be paying attention to the wellbeing of all members of the family.

We shouldn't overstate this. If we pay attention to what is at stake for parents and other family members, that does not mean that we should ignore what is at stake for the child or allow the child to be harmed for the sake of other family members. If there is a serious clash between the interests of the child and of the parents, we should favour the child. Along these lines, the United Nations Convention on the Rights of the Child states that 'In all actions concerning children … the best interests of the child shall be a primary consideration.'[9] Rather, the idea is that we shouldn't ignore that the child is part of a family, and that these decisions affect people other than just the child. Returning to the balancing metaphor that we discussed in Chapter 3, if there is a situation where the benefits and burdens are closely balanced, and it isn't clear which way the scales are leaning, the interests and wishes of parents may tip the balance.

The zone of parental discretion

There are a number of reasons that parents' views and wishes are ethically relevant to decisions about medical treatment for children. If we take those reasons into account, that suggests that whether or not treatment is provided for a child with a given health condition will vary from family to family. Some families may strongly desire treatment, feeling that it would be best for their child, and it will be provided. Other families may feel, in the same circumstance, that that treatment is not the best thing for their child, and treatment will be withheld or stopped.

Situations where treatment might or might not be provided, depending on the family's wishes, represent what Australian ethicist Lynn Gillam and her colleagues call the 'zone of parental discretion'.[10] Discretion here is the idea that parents may decide one way or the other. As she describes it, this is the 'ethically and legally protected space where parents may legitimately make decisions for their children, even if the decisions are … not absolutely the best for them.'[11]

The idea that parents would be consulted about decisions, that they would be an integral part of the decision-making process for children, is hardly controversial. It is, in fact, what happens all the time in the medical care of children all around the world. That includes the most serious and fraught decisions that are ever made – about providing or stopping life support for seriously ill children. It is widely accepted that the right approach to these decisions in most cases involves sharing the decision between professionals and parents.[12]

However, if we think that there is a 'space' where parents' views are important and their wishes will be respected, there must also be an area beyond where parents' wishes are not going to determine whether or not a child has treatment. The more weight that we give to parental interests or autonomy, the wider the range of cases where parents will decide. While there might be agreement internationally that there is a 'zone of parental discretion', there is not as much agreement about how wide this zone is, or where the boundaries of the zone lie. In the Charlie Gard case, the UK courts and doctors clearly felt that Charlie's situation was not one that fell within the zone of discretion. However, other commentators, including ethicists and doctors from the US, felt differently – that this was a decision that parents should be allowed to make, even if we disagree with it.[13] When the European Court of Human Rights considered the Charlie Gard appeal, they assessed whether the balance between the competing interests of child and parents had been struck 'within the margin of appreciation afforded to States in such matters'.[2] This highlights that the court expected and accepted that different states might draw the boundaries of parental discretion in different places.

Where should the boundaries be drawn?

The harm threshold

In Gillam's analysis of parental discretion, she described the limits as set by the 'harm threshold': parents should not be able to make a decision 'if the child is likely to suffer significant harm from the decision'.[11] This builds on previous accounts of decision-making for children by US bioethicists and paediatricians Doug Diekema and Lainie Friedman Ross.[14,15] It also aligns with the much older harm principle articulated by 19th century English philosopher John Stuart Mill: 'The only purpose for which power can be rightfully exercised over any member of a civilized community, against his will, is to prevent harm to others.'[b]

As noted in the first chapter, some of the legal argument in the Charlie Gard case was based on whether a harm threshold should be the legal test for deciding whether to overrule parents who have chosen a treatment alternative. The court ruled that that was not the current standard in UK law around medical treatment (though the judges also noted that, even if such a standard had applied, that it would not have changed their verdict).

However, there is good reason to think that the harm threshold is what should be the basis for overruling parents. To turn the question around: if we think that a particular decision isn't

---

[b]Mill's harm principle implies that a state can limit liberty for the purpose of preventing harm – though does not imply that it must. On Mill's own account, harm might not be enough on its own to justify intervening.[16]

likely to cause significant harm to the child, why should doctors or the courts step in? What business is it of theirs?

Here is an example case that, to our knowledge, has never been tested in a UK court (or any court), but we suggest provides strong support for the harm threshold:

> *Adam is 6 years old. Tragically, at the age of 4 he was involved in a car accident that killed his mother. He suffered severe brain damage and has been left in a persistent vegetative state. Adam's clinical condition has not changed, despite the best available medical care. He lives at home with his father, who, since the death of his wife, has devoted all of his energy to caring for Adam.*
>
> *Adam is dependent on artificial nutrition and hydration provided by a feeding tube (gastrostomy), but does not require any other form of invasive medical treatment to stay alive. His medical treatment is funded by a generous legal settlement that Adam's father was awarded following the accident.*
>
> *The medical consultant caring for Adam has come to the view that Adam will never recover, and that it is not in his best interests to keep him alive. He applies to the court for permission to withdraw artificial feeding. Adam's father is utterly opposed to this plan. He accepts that Adam will likely never improve, but wishes to continue to care for him for Adam's sake, and for the sake of his deceased wife.*

It seems to us unlikely (but not impossible) that a legal case such as the one described would arise. We suspect that few or no medical professionals in a case like this would be willing to go to court to seek withdrawal of artificial feeding against the wishes of a devoted parent. However, it also seems to us that, on the basis of UK law and precedent, the legal verdict in this hypothetical case should be clear. If Adam is genuinely in a persistent vegetative state, then the courts have determined that he would have no interest in continuing medical treatment. His father's wishes about treatment are not thought to be relevant to his interests. As continued artificial feeding is not in Adam's interests, it would be unlawful to continue to provide it. Accordingly, it should be withdrawn.

But if that is a correct interpretation of British law, we suggest that the law is ethically flawed. It would be wrong to withdraw artificial feeding from Adam against his father's objections. While it is plausible that Adam is not benefiting from continued artificial feeding, it is also not harming him.

Should UK law be revised to adopt the harm threshold for disputes about medical treatment? One question is whether it is actually necessary. We have suggested a hypothetical case, where the current legal approach might judge treatment to not be in a child's best interests, though it is not harmful. In practice, though, it seems likely that most if not all cases that reach the court would already cross the harm threshold. As we suggested earlier, it seems highly unlikely that any health professional or NHS trust would embark on legal action to oppose parents unless they felt that what parents were requesting was harmful. We do not actually think it is likely that Adam's case would arise. If that claim is correct, a change in the law would not lead to a change in court decisions. It might be valuable to clarify the ethical basis for overruling parents; however, it wouldn't actually change decisions that are made. The Appeal Court judges in the Gard case suggested that (in their view) the same decision would have been reached in that case whether a harm or best interests test were applied.

Even if there is no harm to the child, there is one potential justification for not acquiescing with parental requests for treatment. In Chapter 4, we discussed in some detail the possibility that providing a particular treatment option would cause indirect harm to other children. Distributive justice considerations may preclude the state continuing to pay for such futile medical treatment.

(That wouldn't apply in the case of Adam because providing artificial nutrition would not deprive any other patients of medical treatment.)

If that is right, then the boundaries of the zone of parental discretion would be determined by these two separate conditions: either where a decision would cause harm to the child or where it would cause harm to others (i.e., through a violation of principles of distributive justice). Of course, if distributive justice is the reason for limiting treatment, it only provides a limit to state-funded treatment. If Adam's father was prepared to meet the costs of providing his artificial nutrition and hydration, there would be no barrier to its provision.

For the rest of this book, we are going to assume that this is the correct ethical basis for overruling parents' decisions about treatment. However, we cannot stop there. We are going to need to do more to decide what counts as enough harm. For example, in Doug Diekema's formulation of the harm threshold, he argues that state intervention is justified if parental refusal of treatment places a child at serious risk of serious preventable harm. But how high a risk is a 'serious risk'? What type or level of harm is 'serious harm'? There may be different answers to those questions in different parts of the world.

Zones of parental discretion and medical tourism

In early 2017, the French supreme court (the Conseil d'Etat) considered an appeal relating to the care of a brain-damaged infant, Marwa Bouchenafa.[17] In France, the Public Health code L1110-5 allows doctors to discontinue treatment without parental consent if they believe it would be of 'no use, disproportionate, or only serving to artificially maintain life without other effect'.[18] Marwa had contracted a severe viral illness of the brain in late 2016 and was left with brain damage and dependent on a ventilator. Doctors planned to withdraw treatment; however, her parents were opposed. A local court and then the supreme court found that there was sufficient uncertainty about Marwa's outlook that the criteria were not met. In particular, the supreme court made a comment about the importance of parental wishes, particularly for young infants:

> 'à défaut de pouvoir rechercher quelle aurait été la volonté de la personne s'agissant d'un enfant de moins d'un an ... l'avis de ses parents, qui s'opposent tous les deux à l'arrêt des traitements, revêt une importance particulière.'
> 'for an infant younger than a year old, in the absence of being able to ascertain what would have been her wishes ... the views of her parents, who are both opposed to withdrawal of treatment, are particularly important.'[19]

This quote suggests that courts in France may give considerably more weight to the wishes of parents than UK courts. That would mean that the zone of parental discretion would potentially be wider in France than in the UK. This probably applies to the US and Australia, where, at least anecdotally, parents are accorded significantly more discretion over medical decisions.

If there is international variation in where the boundaries are drawn for decisions, that could give rise to situations where parents are unable to find doctors prepared to provide treatment in one country, but are able to find some overseas. Perhaps they could embark on a special form of so-called 'medical tourism'? That was, of course, one of the key issues in the Charlie Gard case. It was also raised in the case of Child A, an infant diagnosed with brain death, whose parents wished to take him to Saudi Arabia, and in the case of Ashya King (discussed in the previous chapter).

What should we do in situations like this? Should patients or parents be prevented from accessing treatment overseas?

You might (or might not) be persuaded in the case of experimental medical treatment for Charlie Gard, continued mechanical ventilation for Child A or provision of artificial feeding in the case of Adam. But here are a number of other possible cases:

1. Gender reassignment. A 10-year-old apparently identifies as transgender. His parents have arranged for him to travel to Australia for hormone treatment and surgical gender reassignment.
2. Female genital cutting. A 2-year-old girl's mother had a form of female genital cutting as a young child. Her parents have arranged for travel to Sudan, where a local doctor is prepared to provide the procedure. This involves the surgical removal of her clitoris and oversewing of the vagina.
3. Ashley procedure. The parents of a profoundly cognitively impaired 7-year-old have identified a specialist in the US who is prepared to provide hormone treatment to reduce C's growth, as well as surgery to remove developing breast tissue and her uterus. C's parents hope that these treatments will make C easier to care for.[20]
4. Euthanasia. A 9-year-old boy with a terminal neurodegenerative disorder has progressive neurological decline and is no longer able to communicate. His parents wish to travel to Belgium to access euthanasia.

For medical tourism involving adults, there is some reason to believe that the state should only intervene in an individual's freedom in order to avoid harm to others (that would be the implication of Mill's harm principle mentioned earlier.) If an individual's competent decision to receive medical treatment affects only themselves, why should a government prohibit someone travelling to obtain that treatment, or prosecute them subsequently?

UNLAWFUL CHOICE TOURISM

But focussing on children makes it clearer that there could be strong reasons to prohibit overseas medical choices. In at least some of the previous examples, the parents' decisions to pursue treatment overseas would be illegal. Parents should not be able to get around a law designed to protect children by taking their child overseas. It should not be a defence that, in the overseas country, it is not regarded as harmful to (for example) perform female genital cutting or perform euthanasia.

There are complex issues here around international law and the interaction between different jurisdictions. However, in simple terms, the laws of a country apply to its citizens and provide limits on behaviour, as well as legal protections that apply even when the citizens are beyond the country's borders. In the case of parents taking a child overseas for a prohibited medical option, it seems that the parents could be guilty of a crime in their home country, and that the child should be protected from being the victim of a crime.

One option would be for individuals to renounce their citizenship.[21] That would potentially allow an adult to access options available overseas without being subject to the laws of their original country. It could potentially be thought to apply to children too – though in practice a number of countries (e.g., US, UK) do not allow minors to renounce citizenship until they have reached the age of 16 to 18.

For some highly controversial issues on which a community has divided views, one option would be to specifically allow patients to access that option overseas. For example, the Irish Constitution includes a subsection (focused on the rights of foetuses and on abortion) specifying that women have a right to obtain information about treatment available overseas and have a right to travel. Another compromise is to elect not to prosecute citizens who access prohibited medical options overseas. In the UK, while it remains illegal to do so, there have been no prosecutions of people for helping someone to travel overseas to obtain assisted suicide. It isn't clear, though, that this applies to children. Guidance from the UK Director of Public

Prosecutions implies that prosecution would be more likely in the case of a patient less than 18 years.[22]

If particular medical treatment options for a child are clearly unlawful, and if the prohibitions on those options are valid, it seems justified for doctors and the courts to intervene to prevent parents from travelling to obtain that option. This would seem to apply at least to cases 2 and 4 (earlier).

LEGALLY UNCERTAIN CHOICES TOURISM

But some controversial options may be legally, as well as ethically, grey. It isn't clear what the legal status would be of gender reassignment surgery for a young child in the UK or of the Ashley treatment. If such treatment were requested, court approval might well be sought, and the court would assess whether such treatment were in the best interests of the child. It isn't clear what the decision would be. If the court decided that it would be in the child's best interests, there would be no problem with travel. If the court decided that it would not be in a child's best interests to have gender reassignment or the Ashley procedure, it would then be unlawful to perform those procedures for that child. For example, if parents had gone to court for permission to perform the Ashley procedure, and this had been declined by the court, it would then appear legitimate to stop the parents from travelling with their child in order to circumvent the legal decision. That was the situation for Charlie Gard. After the court had determined that treatment wasn't in his best interests, it would not have been lawful to take him overseas for treatment.

But what about where there hasn't yet been a court decision, no determination either way? If a medical option isn't clearly contrary to the law, and there are qualified overseas health professionals willing to provide a treatment, perhaps doctors shouldn't intervene? (If that is the case, it may suggest that parents would be better to take their children overseas before a court reaches a decision – in case they determine that the option would not be in the child's interests.) However, professional bodies such as the General Medical Council (GMC) (doctors' regulatory body in the UK) often require doctors to notify child protection agencies if they suspect risk of harm, even if not certain. In the case of early gender reassignment surgery or the Ashley treatment, there is a potential risk of harm from the procedures, albeit it is not clear whether that harm is outweighed by the benefits. If doctors learned that a family planned to take a child overseas for the Ashley treatment, they would be justified in notifying child protection authorities of the concern for possible harm. When doctors in the Ashya King case learned that his parents had taken him out of hospital (without apparently knowing how to administer necessary medical treatment), they decided to inform authorities.

The fact that treatment is available overseas will not always mean that treatment should be available in a country of origin. For cases where treatment would be illegal, or legally uncertain, there is a case for preventing medical tourism.

However, there are two ways that the availability of treatment overseas might positively influence treatment disputes in legally uncertain cases. The first possibility is that, where doctors or the courts become aware that treatment is available overseas, they may revise their view about whether or not treatment would be harmful. For example, some infants with the severe chromosomal disorders trisomy 13 or 18 have congenital heart problems. There is controversy within cardiologists and cardiac surgeons about whether surgery should be offered for infants with this condition.[23] Some believe that open heart surgery is not in the best interests of infants with trisomy 13 or 18.[24] However, if a family had identified health professionals overseas who were prepared to provide surgery, it may be possible for the local consultants to speak with the overseas specialists and to review their professional experience of caring for similar patients. Alternatively, the overseas specialist may be able to appear as an expert in a court hearing. That may allay fears about potential harm and make it possible for the family to travel.

The second possibility is that awareness of the range of decisions made overseas (and their outcomes) may help to inform debate about treatment. In some cases, that could encourage health professionals to offer treatment locally so that travel is no longer necessary.

Conclusion

In this chapter, we have identified that parents' wishes or views about treatment are relevant, though parents may be overruled if treatment would be harmful to the child or to other children. We have also started to see that whether or when treatment would be judged to be harmful will be influenced by the values of a society, as well as the views of health professionals. We are going to now specifically focus on the role of agreement and disagreement in evaluating treatment.

References

1. *Great Ormond Street Hospital v Yates & Ors* [2017] EWHC 972 *(Fam)* (11 April 2017).
2. Charles Gard and Others v the United Kingdom: Application No 39793/17: *European Court of Human Rights (First Section)*.
3. Paris, J. J. (2010) Autonomy does not confer sovereignty on the patient: a commentary on the Golubchuk case. *Am J Bioethics*, 10, 54-6.
4. Savulescu, J. & Clarke, S. (2007) Waiting for a miracle … miracles, miraclism, and discrimination. *South Med J*, 100, 1259-62.
5. Savulescu, J. (1998) Two worlds apart: religion and ethics. *J Med Ethics*, 24, 382-4.
6. Castleberry, C. (2017) 'God makes no mistakes': Christian couple in Michigan are charged with manslaughter after they refused jaundice treatment for their newborn daughter. *Daily Mail*. accessed from <http://www.dailymail.co.uk/news/article-4930978/Jaundice-kills-baby-parents-refuse-treatment-her.html>.
7. *An NHS Trust v MB* [2006] 2 F.L.R. 319.
8. *A Local Health Board v Y (A Child) and Others* [2016] *EWHC 206 (Fam)*.
9. United Nations Human rights. (2002). *'Convention on the Rights of the Child.'* from <http://www.ohchr.org/EN/ProfessionalInterest/Pages/CRC.aspx>.
10. Gillam, L. (2010) Children's bioethics and the zone of parental discretion. *Monash Bioeth Rev*, 20, 1-3.
11. Gillam, L. (2015) The zone of parental discretion: An ethical tool for dealing with disagreement between parents and doctors about medical treatment for a child. *Clinical Ethics*, 11, 1-8.
12. Larcher, V., Craig, F., Bhogal, K., Wilkinson, D. & Brierley, J. (2015) Making decisions to limit treatment in life-limiting and life-threatening conditions in children: a framework for practice. *Arch Dis Child*, 100, s1-s23.
13. Shah, S. K., Rosenberg, A. R. & Diekema, D. S. (2017) Charlie Gard and the limits of best interests. *JAMA Pediatr*, 171, 937-938.
14. Diekema, D. S. (2004) Parental refusals of medical treatment: the harm principle as threshold for state intervention. *Theoretical Medicine and Bioethics*, 25, 243-64.
15. Ross, L. F. (1998) *Children, families, and health care decision making*. Oxford, Clarendon Press.
16. Mill, J. S. (1956) *On Liberty*. New York, Bobbs-Merrill.
17. (2017d) *Bébé dans le coma: le Conseil d'Etat ordonne la poursuite des soins de Marwa à Marseille*. Le parisien. accessed from <http://www.leparisien.fr/societe/marseille-le-conseil-d-etat-ordonne-la-poursuite-des-soins-de-la-petite-marwa-08-03-2017-6744171.php>.
18. Pope, T. (2017). 'Marwa Bouchenafa - French Court Orders Clinicians to Treat Baby over Their Objections.' *Medical Futility Blog* from <http://medicalfutility.blogspot.co.uk/2017/03/marwa-bouchenafa-french-court-orders_19.html>.

19. *Conseil d'État*, ordonnance du juge des référés du 8 mars 2017, n° 408146 ECLI:FR:CEORD: 2017:408146.20170308 from <https://www.doctrine.fr/d/CE/2017/CEW408146>.

20. Liao, S. M., Savulescu, J. & Sheehan, M. (2007) The Ashley Treatment: best interests, convenience, and parental decision-making. *Hastings Cent Rep*, 37, 16-20.

21. Cohen, I. (2012) Circumvention tourism. *Cornell Law Review*, 97, 1309.

22. Topping, A. (2009) New assisted suicide guidelines to give 'clear advice' to relatives. *The Guardian*. Accessed from <https://www.theguardian.com/society/2009/sep/23/assisted-suicide-guidelines-legal>.

23. Young, A. A., Simpson, C. & Warren, A. E. (2017) Practices and attitudes of Canadian cardiologists caring for patients with trisomy 18. *Can J Cardiol*, 33, 548-551.

24. Graham, E. M. (2016) Infants with trisomy 18 and complex congenital heart defects should not undergo open heart surgery. *J Law Med Ethics*, 44, 286-91.

Agreeing to Disagree

CHAPTER 7

Dissensus and value pluralism

"'I quite agree with you," said the Duchess; "and the moral of that is—'Be what you would seem to be'—or, if you'd like it put more simply—'Never imagine yourself not to be otherwise than what it might appear to others that what you were ...'"

Alice's Adventures in Wonderland, Lewis Carroll

'I am not deciding ... whether the respective decisions of the doctors on the one hand or the parents on the other are reasonable decisions.'[1]

JUSTICE HOLMAN, re MB 2006

In earlier chapters, we identified some core areas of disagreement around life and death decisions for seriously ill patients. For example, there are differing views about what it means for treatment to be futile, what chance of improvement would be too low to provide treatment, when a patient is harmed by treatment, when treatment would lack objective benefits, when the evidence is enough to show that treatment works or doesn't work, how to evaluate when scarce or expensive treatment should not be provided and where the boundaries of parental discretion should lie. We (the authors) have different views on some of these questions, and, as the first chapters illustrated, we have also disagreed about how to apply these ethical questions in the case of Charlie Gard.

Does this disagreement matter, though? In this chapter, we are going to explore some of the ethical implications of diverging ethical viewpoints. Ultimately, we suggest that disagreement can help us to identify a range of options that patients or families may pursue. We will start though, by focussing our sights on one potential view about treatment decisions that places great emphasis on agreement.

Consensus

Many professional guidelines suggest that health professionals need to reach consensus before making a decision to stop life-sustaining medical treatment. We could call this the 'consensus' view about treatment limitation. (We will return to the opposite sort of question (about providing treatment) shortly.) For example, in 2003 the Australasian Intensive Care Society endorsed the need for professional consensus: 'Any decision to withdraw or limit treatment first requires the *consensus* of the intensive care team and the primary medical or surgical team.'[2]

In the same year, UK Intensive Care Society guidelines stated: 'Ideally, there should be *consensus* among the entire clinical team who have been heavily involved in the patient's care, that it is appropriate to withhold or withdraw aggressive treatment.... Unanimity is desirable but may be unobtainable.'[3] More recently, the UK medical regulatory body, the General Medical Council (GMC), noted: 'You should aim to reach a *consensus* about what treatment and care would be of overall benefit to a patient who lacks capacity.'[4]

'Consensus' isn't defined in these documents. The word is originally derived from Latin (*consentire*, literally: to feel or think together).[5] The professional guidelines vary in how much emphasis they

TABLE 7.1 ■ Levels of agreement in decisions

		Proportion favoring ultimate course of action
Consensus decisions	Unanimous	100%
	Near unanimous	E.g., >90%
	Majority view	>50%
Nonconsensus decisions		
	Largest group (non-majority)	<50%
	Minority view	<50%

place on agreement. They encompass a spectrum from consensus being mandatory (Australasian Intensive Care Society), through to it being merely something to aspire to (GMC). We might also note that there are different degrees of agreement that could be labelled 'consensus' (Table 7.1). At one end of the spectrum lies uniform agreement. (The Australian and UK intensive care guidelines appear to use consensus in this way.) Another Australian guideline, which strongly promotes a consensus-building model, notes that it may be possible to reach decisions if one person disagrees:

> 'In circumstances where one team member is in disagreement with the others, the team as a whole should ... seek the opinions of professionals from the same discipline as the disagreeing member. In the event that support for this position cannot be found, it may be appropriate for the dissenting member not to continue being involved in the treating team.'[6]

At the other end of the spectrum, some people might regard decisions supported by the majority (i.e., >50%) as also being a type of consensus.

One reason why agreement might be thought important or necessary is because of the seriousness of decisions about life support. The 'sanctity of life' principle is strongly endorsed by many societies.[7] This does not mean that life must always be prolonged.[8] However, it does potentially mean that medical decisions to stop (or not start) life-sustaining treatment should be taken cautiously and only where there is certainty that it is the right thing to do.

A second reason to seek consensus is its practical and psychological value. It is likely to be helpful for families to know that health professionals all agree that life-sustaining treatment is not in the patient's best interests. Professional agreement (and a clear recommendation) might avoid families feeling as if they are carrying the full burden of decisions and leave them less likely to feel guilty for a decision to discontinue treatment. On the other hand, professional disagreement could be distressing for families.[9,10] It would potentially make it less likely that families would agree to treatment being withdrawn or limited.

Finally, consensus may be valuable for the health professionals involved. It would potentially help them to feel confident in a decision not to provide treatment.[11] It could reduce legal vulnerability. Professionals are sometimes concerned about the possibility that a controversial decision would end up with them in trouble with the law.[12] If all of a doctor's professional colleagues are agreed that it is ethical to withdraw or withhold treatment, it would appear much less likely that the doctor would be prosecuted, or that prosecution would be successful. As we saw previously, the Bolam standard expresses this view in law.

However, if we think that consensus is necessary before doctors can stop life support, or that agreement is ideal, the disagreement that we have described in this book poses a serious problem. Without a common answer to the questions listed at the start of this chapter, it may not be possible for all professionals to agree. If unanimous or near-unanimous consensus is required, end-of-life decisions could be held hostage by the most conservative or cautious decision makers. One or two professionals with strong views against limitation of treatment could exert a veto over decisions, even if the family holds quite different views.

We have mentioned in earlier chapters that life and death medical decisions are based not only on medical facts, but also on values. There is clear evidence from a large number of studies internationally that physicians vary in the values that they apply to end-of-life decisions and, consequently, in the decisions they make.[13,14] Decisions are influenced by physician gender, age, religion and personal views.[15] Studies have shown that doctors desire fewer life-sustaining interventions than patients do,[16–18] and do not necessarily share patients' religious and cultural values.[19] Doctors' own preferences for life-sustaining treatment appear to influence their perception or assessment of what the patient would want.[20] One study used a simulation of adult ICU end-of-life decision-making: 27 doctors were given medical information and a chance to interview an elderly cancer patient and his wife. They were asked to make a decision about providing life-sustaining treatment. There was considerable variation in the decisions made. Less than half of the participating doctors treated the patient according to his wishes, despite the patient and his wife having clear, stable preferences about intensive care.[21] A requirement that health teams reach consensus before deciding to limit treatment may frequently mean that the values of physicians are imposed on the patient and the family.

Next, while seeking medical consensus may reflect understandable caution about making decisions that would lead to death, it is not clear that this is the only way to ensure that safe and appropriate decisions are made. Indeed, it seems likely that this approach would prolong potentially burdensome treatment and merely delay inevitable death in at least some patients.

Finally, while there might be psychological benefits for families if doctors have reached consensus, that does not mean that treatment must continue where consensus does not exist and there are different views within the medical team. Families could (in some circumstances) feel excluded if they learn that discussions about the ethics of treatment for their child have occurred in their absence. At least some families would benefit from acknowledgment of the ethical complexity of decisions and the importance of their own perspective.

Most importantly, the fact that there is consensus does not necessarily mean that such decisions are right. People are corrigible, or capable of making mistakes. These decisions are complex, requiring sophisticated deployment of ethical concepts and principles in an impartial manner. Doctors, patients, nurses and families are unlikely to be ethical experts and may not even be aware of the relevant concepts and their interplay.

Instead of trying to achieve agreement, we propose that professionals should acknowledge and accept disagreement in ethically complex decisions.

Doctors and parents (and adult patients) bring a range of different values to end-of-life decisions. These values lead individuals to make different decisions. There is uncertainty, for example, about the effectiveness of treatment, or the patient's quality of life if they survive.

Moreover, there is moral uncertainty about how to weigh up the risks and benefits of treatment. Doctors should not set themselves the impossible goal of seeking the single and only right course of action. Instead, they need to examine whether there are a range of reasonable courses of action over which patients/families may exercise choice. It is a mistake to think that there is always one course, and that a group of clinicians can identify it.

Here, we clearly take a different perspective from the judge in the MB case (quoted at the start of the chapter). Justice Holman rejected the idea that his role was to assess the reasonableness of the different views or treatment options. Instead, he claimed that the judge's role was to apply an 'objective test' and to reach an independent and objective verdict about what would be in the child's best interests. While that is undoubtedly a correct interpretation of the UK legal framework for decisions, as a point of practical ethics it is more questionable. We might believe there is some objectively right answer to ethical dilemmas. However, for all the reasons that we have outlined earlier, it is doubtful that there is an objective test available to us that can always answer the question of what would be best for a child in all circumstances. Of course, there may be some situations where one course of action would be clearly better for a child, or where what is being requested by parents is harmful. However, in other cases, there will be reasonable disagreement. Where there is such disagreement, it is wrong for judges or doctors to impose their own particular view about what would be best and override reasonable requests from parents or families.

To summarise, we have argued against the view that professionals should reach consensus before making a decision to stop life support. Decisions about providing or not providing life-sustaining treatment are ethically complex. We do not think that there is a need for professionals to reach agreement before deciding to limit treatment. On the contrary, as long as the decision would be lawful, dissensus would be enough. We have referred to this idea as the 'reasonable dissensus' view about limiting treatment[22]:

> Reasonable dissensus view about limiting treatment: Treatment limitation may be discussed with families and may proceed where at least one member of the treating team who is aware of the relevant clinical facts, after adequate reflection and discussion, would endorse such a decision (and would be prepared to take over the care of the patient if they are not the responsible clinician).

It may be helpful to illustrate how this might work. One of us (DW) works in a newborn ICU where there are 10 consultant specialists. Long-term patients in the ICU are discussed in regular weekly senior team meetings where most consultants are present. For patients who have involvement from other medical specialists, where there are difficult or contentious treatment decisions, we convene ad hoc multidisciplinary meetings with senior representatives of each team. Here is a type of case that we have faced on more than one occasion.

> *A newborn infant, Sean, has breathing difficulties after birth and is urgently intubated (put on life support) and brought to the ICU.[a] He is found to have a number of congenital abnormalities, including problems affecting his heart and lungs. If Sean is to survive, he will need major surgery to correct a hole in his diaphragm. Sean has some further tests that reveal an underlying genetic problem. Case reports of other infants with this problem suggest that some infants with this problem die early in life, while those who survive can have a range of long-term developmental problems that might be severe, or might be less severe. Some members of the team question whether Sean should undergo major surgery for his lung problem, or whether he should instead be provided with palliative care and allowed to die.*

According to the consensus view, to decide not to provide intensive life-sustaining treatment (surgery for the hole in the diaphragm in this case), there would need to be support from at least half of the 10 consultants (as well as the other specialists involved) before discussing the option of limiting treatment with families. On more stringent interpretations of the consensus view, all or almost all of the specialists would need to agree with a decision to limit treatment before approaching the family (i.e., 9 or 10 neonatal specialists plus other specialist consultants involved).

However, we have rejected the consensus view of treatment limitation. This level of agreement is too stringent; it may not be possible, for one thing. But more importantly, consensus is not required for medically and ethically complex decisions where there can be a range of

[a]This is a composite case.

different reasonable views. On the contrary, treatment limitation should be an option if there is reasonable dissensus. If at least one of the neonatal consultants or other specialists believe that it is potentially in the child's best interests to withdraw or withhold treatment, it would be ethical to discuss that option with the family and to proceed with the decision if the family agree.

In our definition of reasonable dissensus, we stipulated two important conditions. The dissenting view must persist after adequate discussion and reflection. Imagine a situation where some specialists are in favour of limiting treatment because they are not aware of all the relevant facts. They might believe, for example, that the outcomes for infants with this genetic problem are universally poor, while the most recent published data do not support this. Such factual misunderstanding does not provide evidence of reasonable disagreement. If that were the reason why some specialists had a different view about treatment, we would expect the dissenter to revise their view once appraised of the latest evidence.

We also proposed that the dissenting doctors would need to be prepared to take over the care of the patient (as well as taking responsibility for the decision to limit treatment). This requires a high level of commitment to decisions and would require nontreating consultants to take the decision just as seriously as the treating consultant. This can't be an 'armchair' opinion. This condition would also potentially address concerns related to conscientious objection. If the current treating consultant is unhappy with the idea of not performing surgery, they could potentially ask those members of the team who do support withdrawal or withholding of treatment to take over discussion with the family and management.[b]

The model that we have described does not mention other members of the healthcare team who may or may not support limiting treatment. For example, it might be that all of the consultants in the team want to continue treatment for a child, while some of the bedside nurses or junior doctors looking after a patient are concerned about the amount of pain or discomfort that a child is experiencing and believe that it is time to move to palliative care. In that sort of situation, the views of nursing or junior medical staff are important. When specialists discuss treatment for a child, they should seek out the views of other members of the team. They should make sure that there are opportunities for all members of the clinical team to express their views. Where other people articulate serious concerns about the wisdom of continuing treatment, that should lead the specialists involved to reflect on their own views and consider whether treatment limitation should actually be an option to be discussed with parents.

We suggested that one reason to seek consensus is because that is perceived as safer for patients. What safeguards would there be for decisions if we adopted a different threshold and allowed treatment to be withdrawn even if professionals disagree amongst themselves? There are several conceivable. Decisions would still need to be consistent with the prevailing law on end-of-life decisions. The responsible consultant, on the dissensus view, would remain legally responsible for their decision. Indeed, given that peers take a different view, the physician would potentially hold a greater personal responsibility for action. This would mean that they would need to take additional care to justify their decision and to clearly document their reasons for doing so.[c] Furthermore, we could build in additional processes for decisions made in the

---

[b]We have, however, argued elsewhere that in this sort of situation, the treating consultant should usually <u>not</u> conscientiously object even if s/he has a right to do so. Once it is clear that there are different reasonable views about treatment, and one or more colleagues would support a decision to limit treatment, we have argued that the doctor should set aside his or her own personal beliefs and provide the option to the family.[23]

[c]On this basis, a decision reached in the absence of consensus might be safer than one reached with mutual agreement. Collective decisions can sometimes give an illusion of security, and it is possible for groups to make decisions together than they would not individually endorse.[24]

absence of agreement. For example, ethics consultation might be mandatory in such situations. However, the aim of such consultation would not be to achieve collective agreement – rather to ensure that the decision is consistent with prevailing policy or law, that all appropriate factors have been considered and that the proposed limitation of treatment is a reasonable course of action.[d]

Reasonable dissensus

We have proposed that reasonable disagreement would make it ethical to limit life-sustaining treatment – if parents agree. That might not seem relevant to the main topic of this book. The Charlie Gard case and the other cases mentioned in this book have all been situations where parents do not agree and do not wish to limit treatment.

However, reasonable dissensus could also be applied to decisions about *providing* life-sustaining treatment.

> Reasonable dissensus view about providing medical treatment: Treatment provision may be discussed with families and may proceed (*) where at least one member of the treating team who is aware of the relevant clinical facts, after adequate reflection and discussion, would endorse such a decision (and would be prepared to take over the care of the patient if they are not the responsible clinician).

This appears to be a symmetrical version of the view about limiting treatment we described earlier (we will discuss one important modification marked (*) shortly).

In the newborn ICU, one of us (DW) has frequently faced situations where the majority of consultants have felt that continued treatment for a gravely ill infant is not in the child's best interests. For example:

> *A newborn infant, Sian, is born extremely prematurely, stabilised and brought to the neonatal ICU.[e] She develops a series of complications and has progressively worsening lung problems. After several months of treatment, she is now full-term. For the last few weeks she has been receiving maximal levels of support from a breathing machine and has not improved, despite all available treatment. X-rays of her lungs show severe cystic lung damage. She is felt to be too unstable for a tracheostomy, while the paediatric ICU are reluctant to accept transfer as they believe that she will not survive. Her parents are opposed to withdrawal of treatment.*

In cases like this, our experience has been that sometimes the majority of the clinical team have felt that life-sustaining treatment is harmful to the infant and should not continue. Yet a minority of consultants have disagreed. They have cited cases in their past experience of infants improving despite apparently dire prognosis. Or they have felt that it would not be wrong to continue treatment because Sian's possible pain and discomfort from treatment could be relieved with drugs. Alternatively, they may have agreed that Sian was not likely to survive but felt that it was inevitable that she would 'declare herself' in the coming days or weeks, deteriorating further and dying despite maximal treatment. That would spare parents a decision that they could not accept. If the child will die in any case, it could be a worse outcome overall if the clinical team attempt to impose a decision on parents (for example, by taking the parents to court).

[d]Ethics committees vary in their legal expertise, and in some institutions legal questions are dealt with by a separate process.[25]
[e]This is a composite of real cases.

Where there is reasonable disagreement about what would be in the best interests of a child or would be harmful to the child, we suggest that continuing treatment should potentially be an option. We propose that clinical teams should not, in this circumstance, impose unilateral decisions on Sian's parents, or embark upon legal action.

To some, that conclusion might seem obvious. It may be that this is already how clinicians deal with decisions about providing treatment. It is, after all, relatively unlikely that hospitals would seek a court order in a situation where some in the hospital are prepared to provide treatment that the parents are requesting. The child could just be transferred to the care of a consultant who is willing to treat. It is only when all of the relevant consultants are opposed to continuing treatment that a court might become involved.

However, once we look beyond the walls of a single hospital, the implications of the dissensus model are more significant. It may be that all of the specialists in one hospital are opposed to providing treatment in the case of Sian, but what if there are specialists elsewhere who are in favour of treatment? What if those specialists have different qualifications or expertise? What if they are based in another country? Does that change whether or not treatment should be provided?

One of the basic philosophical ideas underlying the dissensus approach is that of pluralism. There are different types of pluralism described within philosophy. For example, at a fundamental level, some have argued for metaphysical pluralism – the idea that there are different types of fundamental essence or substance in the universe, or even that there is more than one reality. Epistemological pluralism refers to the idea that there is not one consistent set of truths about the world – rather there are different ways of perceiving, knowing and understanding the world. Moral or value pluralism refers to the idea that there are different ultimate sources of value. This view, particularly associated with the Oxford philosopher Isaiah Berlin, is often linked to the idea that values are incommensurable. They are like apples and oranges. There is no way of directly comparing them; for example, one orange isn't equivalent to a particular number of apples. Where there is a conflict between different values, there may not be any way of objectively ordering or ranking alternative courses of action. Finally, political pluralism refers to the idea that within any society, there will be a diversity of value systems and a diversity of views about how to live. As a consequence, negotiation, tolerance and compromise are necessary.

Metaphysical pluralism is probably not terribly relevant to practical decisions about life support. Epistemological pluralism might be relevant. In Chapter 5, we discussed the different approaches to identifying and evaluating evidence about treatments. Value pluralism is obviously highly relevant because of the range of competing values involved in end-of-life decisions. It is this form of pluralism that we are primarily concerned with in this book. However, even for those who are inclined to think that there is a single correct way of evaluating evidence, or a single relevant value that applies to medical treatment, there is the further problem that, in the real world, there is no way to achieve uniform agreement about that. Political pluralism is, it would seem, inescapable.

It is worth distinguishing pluralism from 'relativism'. Sometimes people are drawn to think that values, perceptions or views are relative to the observer. There are neither correct nor incorrect answers, since judgments depend on the individual. There are just different answers. Pluralism also endorses more than one value, value system or viewpoint. There can be more than one correct answer. However, there can also be one or more incorrect answers. Pluralism does not mean supporting any value or any value system that someone happens to support. It does not mean that all answers are equally acceptable. Isaiah Berlin famously rejected the suggestion that accepting pluralism meant that 'anything goes':

> 'I am not a relativist; I do not say "I like my coffee with milk and you like it without; I am in favor of kindness and you prefer concentration camps" – each of us with his own values, which cannot be overcome or integrated'.[26]

The dissensus view that we have described is based on pluralism – not on relativism. Not all cases of disagreement would mean that treatment should be provided. In our account of dissensus, we specified that disagreement must be reasonable. Let us imagine, for example, that in a case like that of Sian, it becomes clear that, while all the consultants at this hospital are opposed to treatment, the family has found a specialist elsewhere who believes that treatment would be in Sian's best interests. That was exactly the situation in the Gard, Bowen and Simms cases. One key issue is whether this disagreement is reasonable.

When we discussed treatment limitation, we proposed some practical conditions that would help assess whether the disagreement is reasonable or unreasonable. These conditions do not guarantee that disagreement is reasonable; they do, however, make it more likely that the dissenting view is reasonable. We will later suggest some additional criteria for reasonableness.

The first condition was that the dissenting clinician must be aware of the relevant clinical facts, and their view must persist after adequate reflection and discussion. If we became aware, for example, that the specialist who has provided an opinion in favour of treatment for Sian had made an assessment without knowledge of Sian's specific circumstances, that might call into question whether his or her view about treatment was adequately informed.

In the real case of Charlie Gard, the judge appeared to give less weight to the views of the US specialist, Professor Hirano, because of an impression that he had reached his view about treatment without being aware of important factors that the clinicians treating Charlie felt were relevant.

In the final High Court hearing, the legal team for the hospital called into question the credibility of the views of Professor Hirano on this basis:

'On 13 July he stated that not only had he not visited the hospital to examine Charlie but in addition, he had not read Charlie's contemporaneous medical records or viewed Charlie's brain imaging or read all of the second opinions about Charlie's condition (obtained from experts all of whom had taken the opportunity to examine him and consider his records) or even read the Judge's decision made on 11 April.'[27]

Justice Francis made a strong claim in the final hearing about the importance of seeing the patient:

'It seems to me to be a remarkably simple proposition that if a doctor is to give evidence to this court about the prospect of effective treatment in respect of a child … that Dr should see the patient before the court can sensibly rely upon his evidence.' (para 12)[28]

However, we cannot necessarily discount a view that has been reached based on only partial information. It may be that examining the patient or knowing the additional facts would not change someone's mind; they may still be prepared to support treatment. In the first Gard hearing, the specialist's view about treatment persisted after he had been made aware of test results and discussed Charlie's condition with the Great Ormond Street doctors:

'I appreciate how unwell he is. His EEG is very severe. I think he is in the terminal stage of his illness. I can appreciate your position. I would just like to offer what we can. It is unlikely to work, but the alternative is that he will pass away.' (para 127)[29]

We have disagreed ourselves over whether Hirano's view was reasonable. One of us (DW) believes it wasn't because Hirano had not physically reviewed Charlie until July. The other (JS) believes it was reasonable because he was provided with all clinical information available, together with relevant test results. It was in fact Hirano who requested a further brain scan before giving an opinion in the first hearing. Seeing the patient in such a circumstance, Julian believed, would yield no other evidence that could sway the opinion. Clearly, whether dissensus is reasonable is a value judgment over which people can disagree.

Perhaps where there is even disagreement about whether there is reasonable disagreement we should look for 'metadissensus' – this would be looking for the spread of views amongst experts about the disagreement itself. Most experts agreed with DW. But two other experts – Professor Peter Singer and Professor Raanan Gillon – agreed with JS. Is this enough? Again, that is a value judgment.

Ultimately, someone has to decide what will be done and that is, in the current UK system, the judge. However, what we should expect is a degree of ethical humility and a willingness to admit of reasonable disagreement. Most importantly, we should hope that judges will recognise that these are as much, if not more, value rather than factual judgments, and acknowledge that reasonable value pluralism can exist.

In another case of desired experimental treatment (for an adult patient with acquired brain injury), it was claimed that an expert (offering treatment) had not examined the patient or reviewed his medical records.[30] Yet, in that instance, the expert's opinion was not rejected. The judge ruled provisionally in favour of allowing treatment, on condition that the expert reviews the medical records for the patient, undertakes a full assessment in person and provides a written report indicating whether he still recommended treatment. So, views reached on the basis of incomplete information don't have to be completely discounted.

The second condition that we proposed as part of the reasonable dissensus view was that the specialist would have to be prepared to take over the care of the patient. That was designed, in part, to test the genuineness or conviction of a dissenter. Imagine, for example, that there is disagreement about major cosmetic surgery for a child. If a surgeon expressed a view that surgery should be an option, but then declined to perform the surgery himself or herself, we might question the credibility of their view. It is also designed to avoid a situation where clinicians who are convinced that treatment would not be in a child's best interests are forced to provide that treatment. The child could be transferred into the care of the specialist who is supportive of treatment.

This condition would restrict dissenting views to medical specialists who are actually able to provide treatment. That appears to be important in one way: it guarantees that they have a relevant type and level of technical expertise. (It would prevent a situation, for example, where a dermatologist is opining about cardiac surgery, or a geriatrician is providing a view about obstetric care.) However, when children require care from a multidisciplinary team, specialists might provide support for elements of care within their remit. In the Gard case, Professor Hirano indicated that he would be prepared to provide nucleoside therapy but would defer to intensive care specialists to make a decision about provision of life support.[29]

We might wonder, though, whether this condition is too restrictive. We have explored in some detail the ethical complexity of decisions about best interests and experimental treatment. Yet, if we are determining whether treatment is a reasonable option based on the views of medical specialists, one concern is that this reduces decisions to a medical or even a technical question. In the Gard case, some of the media commentary was critical of a court process that appeared to be overly deferential to medical experts. While knowledge of medical facts is important, decisions about life-sustaining treatment are also clearly dependent on ethical values and ethical evaluation. Medical expertise does not guarantee ethical expertise.

There are two opposite problems that could arise from a dissensus approach to providing medical treatment.

PROBLEM 1

First, there might be situations where no medical experts are prepared to support treatment – but they should. Here is a possible example: in 2016, the High Court in England and Wales heard the case of JS, a terminally ill teenager who had requested cryopreservation after her body had died, in the hope that, in the future, it might be possible for her to be revived.[31] Cryopreservation (also called cryonics) is a novel and controversial procedure. At the time when JS's case was being discussed, there were commercial companies offering cryopreservation in the US and in Russia. The hospital in that case were supportive of JS's wishes. However, we could imagine another case, where health professionals were opposed to the cryopreservation procedure. (The hospital wrote to the court after JS's death expressing deep misgivings about the conduct and expertise of those who had performed her cryopreservation.[f]) To our knowledge, there are no registered medical specialists in the UK who are involved in cryonics. The preservation procedures for patients in the UK are undertaken by non–medically trained volunteers. A full discussion of the ethical issues around cryopreservation would take us outside the scope of this book. However, there are strong ethical arguments to think that cryopreservation would be a reasonable option after death. First, in some situations (as was the case for JS), knowledge that they were going to be cryopreserved might provide considerable solace and psychological benefit to a dying patient. Second, given that the preservation procedures occur after death has been declared, they cannot cause any pain or harm to the patient himself or herself. Third, if at some distant point in the future there were a possibility of the patient being resuscitated (and having their medical condition cured), that would offer an enormous potential benefit to the patient. Thinking back to our 'weighing' analogy for best interests, this is a situation where the chance of benefit might be miniscule but it might be seen by some as a gamble worth taking given no negatives on the other side.

For cryopreservation, there are potential downsides for other people (for example, the effect on hospital staff or the cost of treatment). There have also been suggested negatives – for example, the possibility of being revived to experience significant physical suffering, or alienation at living in a world in which all familiar people or objects no longer exist. Again, our aim here isn't to settle the question of cryopreservation – rather to suggest that it could be an example of a potentially reasonable option that is nevertheless not supported by any medical specialists. If that were true, then there are two options. The first is that health professionals take into account and try to understand the reasons why patients are requesting treatment. They should be prepared to have an open mind and consider whether they should revise their own views. (In the case of JS, the hospital team did actually support JS's wishes, despite their reservations.)

The second possibility is that we could consider whether some treatments need to be provided by medical specialists. In the case of cryonics, as noted, the procedures are performed by trained (but not medically trained) volunteers.

Another highly relevant example would be that of a request for alternative (nonconventional/non–scientifically proven) medicine. We might imagine a child who is dying from end-stage cancer after exhausting all conventional medical treatments. The child's parents might wish to pursue an alternative medicine, for example, a homeopathic or naturopathic remedy. We shouldn't expect or require alternative medicine to be provided by a conventional medical

---

[f]On JS's last day, her mother is said to have been preoccupied with the post-mortem arrangements at the expense of being fully available to JS. The voluntary organisation is said to have been under-equipped and disorganised, resulting in pressure being placed on the hospital to allow procedures that had not been agreed. Although the preparation of JS's body for cryogenic preservation was completed, the way in which the process was handled caused real concern to the medical and mortuary staff.'[31]

specialist for a child to be allowed to receive this alternative medicine. We will, therefore, need some additional criteria for determining the reasonableness of treatment requests. We will return to those shortly.

PROBLEM 2

The second problem is the opposite one. There might be specialists willing to provide treatment, but that does not guarantee that their reasoning is sound. We have already suggested that ethical expertise doesn't always come with medical expertise. We can't assume that, just because some professionals are prepared to provide treatment, it would be reasonable to do so.

Disagreement between health professionals about treatment for a child provides some evidence that there may be more than one reasonable option. However, it does not (on its own) prove that. We need an additional basis for assessing this.

Reasonableness

What does it mean for a decision or a view to be reasonable? Sometimes people are inclined to use the word to refer to views or opinions with which they agree. We might find ourselves nodding as we read a newspaper article and comment that it seems 'very reasonable'. Or we might complain of someone after an argument that 'he was being unreasonable!'. But if we used the word that way, there could be no sense in which there could be 'reasonable disagreement'. If we are trying to determine whether or not a proposed course of treatment is reasonable, we must have in mind something more like the dictionary definition: treatment that is 'in accordance with reason'.

A full account of what it means to reason is beyond the scope of this book. Like 'best interests' and 'harm', it may be the sort of evaluative concept that can, itself, be interpreted in a range of different plausible ways. However, here are some characteristics that speak in favour of a view being reasonable (or, alternatively, in favour of it being unreasonable).

REASONING PROCESS

First, we can think of the reasoning process that has gone into a decision. For something to be 'reason-able' – it must be able to be articulated or defended or justified in terms of reasons, and those reasons must count in favour of the decision. Imagine that a specialist offered to provide treatment for a child, but when asked why they felt treatment would benefit the child, they reply 'I just do'. In that case, it seems that the decision is lacking sufficient reason or justification. In another example, in Chapter 6 we imagined that the adult Colin Giles wanted to undergo experimental treatment because he liked the name of the drug, or thought that the doctor offering the treatment looked attractive. In this case, Colin can offer reasons for his choice – but they do not seem to count in favour of treatment in any meaningful way. His justifications do not seem reasonable. These are explanatory but not justificatory (or normative) reasons. Of course, even if Colin can't give us good reasons for his choice, that doesn't necessarily make it an unreasonable option. If we reflect on it, we may find that there are reasons that could be given, and that could justify the option. It could still be a reasonable decision (though Colin has not engaged with those reasons in reaching his decision).

REASON-SENSITIVE

Second, for a view to be reasonable, it must be sensitive to the justifying reasons and facts. If the facts or evidence change, and those facts affect the reasons given in favour of the decision, we would expect someone to potentially change their mind. Someone whose view is revisable, and who would be prepared to make a different decision if the evidence changed, is expressing a view that is, on the face of it, eminently reasonable. Conversely, if someone reaches a view but refuses to reconsider that decision when faced with evidence, that appears to undermine or refute the reasons that they gave – their view appears to be unreasonable.

We can all think of examples from our experience where someone's disagreement appears to be unreasonable in this way. You are having an argument with a friend and they express a strong view. You cite some evidence against your friend's view, but they are unwilling to change their mind. Presented with contrary evidence, the friend immediately rejects the credibility of that evidence. Or they may seek instead to provide a new alternative argument in favour of their view. Neither of those strategies, in themselves, proves that their view is unreasonable. The evidence (in favour of your own view) might be flawed. There might be more than one independent argument or reason in favour of their view. However, sometimes we gain the impression that, no matter what evidence is presented, or what argument is advanced, your friend will not change their mind. That seriously calls into question the reasonableness of their view.

On this basis, one way of testing the reasonableness of different points of view would be to ask experts what evidence would change their view about treatment for a child. For example, in the Gard case, the professionals at Great Ormond Street might have been asked what evidence would make them feel that treatment would be in Charlie's interests. The US expert could have been asked the opposite question. Would he ever refuse to provide treatment that parents have requested (and can pay for)? In fact, Hirano did later change his view about the reasonableness of treatment when muscle scans showed advanced damage.

We might call into question the reasonableness of a view if an expert were unable to give any situation or evidence that would change their view. Alternatively, the expert might propose evidence or situations that appear impossible to obtain or completely unrealistic. Again, that would potentially make their view less reasonable.

Of course, it might be the case that someone's views about treatment are based on strongly held values that aren't dependent on particular facts. For example, someone might hold a strong belief in the value of parental autonomy and believe that parents' views about treatment should always be respected. This leads to a third characteristic feature for a reasonable view about treatment.

UNACCEPTABLE REASONS

Parental autonomy

For a view to be reasonable, it must be able to be expressed in terms of the right sort of reasons. We argued previously that reasonable pluralism means accepting a range of views and values, though it does not mean accepting just any value. To express this more pointedly, a reasonable view about treatment cannot be justified on the basis of reasons that are judged to be unacceptable by wider society.

This argument might seem to be circular – we judge a view to be unreasonable because it is based on unreasonable values. However, it does not have to be circular. There may be good independent reasons to exclude particular values from consideration.

We have identified one of these already. Someone has a right to believe, and to express the view, that parents should always have the final say in decisions about medical treatment for a child. However, as discussed in Chapter 6, most societies have considered and rejected that point of view. Parents do not own their children. They are not infallible. They are not always well motivated. Their decisions sometimes risk serious harm to their children. They should not be allowed to refuse definitely beneficial treatment, like treatment for newborn jaundice.

For all of those reasons, we do not think that parents have unlimited discretion about decisions to provide or withhold medical treatment for a child. They do have discretion to decide between reasonable treatment options. However, we can't count a treatment option as being reasonable just because someone is prepared to provide it (and their reason for this is because they believe that parents should always decide). That would be self-defeating and would not make any sense at all.

Sanctity of life

Through much of this book, we have been focussing on questions about continuing life-sustaining medical treatment. Another important value that might justify a particular view about treatment would be based on the value of continued life. For example, someone might hold a strong 'sanctity of life' view. They believe that it is always in a patient's best interests to have their life prolonged, or they might hold the related view that it is never ethical to withdraw life-sustaining treatment. However, on a similar basis to the view about parental autonomy, these do not seem to be acceptable reasons for judging treatment to be a reasonable option. Within societies like Australia, UK, Canada and the US, debate, ethical analysis and legal principles have rejected these views about life-sustaining treatment, at least where the patient or surrogate has agreed that treatment should not be prolonged. In the UK (and in other countries, such as France), societies have come to the stronger conclusion that there are situations where life should not be prolonged even if the patient would have wanted treatment to continue, or the family are requesting that treatment. In those societies, it would not make any sense to count in favour of the reasonableness of providing treatment a view based on a strong sanctity of life ethic.

Here, there may be some divergence between different countries, and we may find pertinent the question that we identified earlier about the location of experts who are offering to support treatment. It may be, for example, that some countries consider the strong sanctity of life view to be acceptable. For example, it is not considered legal to withdraw continuous life-sustaining treatment in Israel.[32] Other countries may not allow withdrawal of treatment without parental agreement. In those countries, it clearly would be regarded as reasonable to continue treatment in a case like that of Charlie Gard.

Evidence of international variation in approach should give policy makers some reason to consider whether their own approach is the right one. It might lead countries to revise their policies. However, where a society has already concluded that it is not always ethical to continue medical treatment, even if strongly desired by patients or requested by families, a view that treatment should be provided based on a strong sanctity of life ethic would not count as reasonable and cannot count in favour of providing treatment.

Religious values?

The strong sanctity of life is particularly associated with certain religious views. That raises the question of whether views in favour of (or against) treatment that are based on religious values would count as reasonable or unreasonable.

One response might be that, where medical experts are asked to provide a view on the reasonableness of medical treatment options (either withdrawal or provision of treatment), they are being asked specifically because of their medical expertise, rather than their theological expertise. If we imagine, for example, a neurologist who provided a view (on the basis of their personal religious view) that treatment should continue for patients who meet criteria for brain death, there might be a question mark about the relevance of their view. Perhaps their view would not be counted as reasonable? We might think similarly about a Jehovah's Witness haematologist who professed a view that transfusions should be withheld at parental request.

In some of the UK court cases, there has been explicit discussion about whether parents' religious views could be included in an assessment of the best interests of the child. For example, in the case of MB, Justice Holman dismissed the relevance of parents' religious views for an assessment of a child's best interests:

> 'This case concerns a child who must himself be incapable, by reason of his age, of any religious belief. An objective balancing of his own best interests cannot be affected by whether a parent happens to adhere to one particular belief, or another, or none. I have the utmost respect for the father's religious faith and belief, and for the faith of Islam which he practises and professes. But I regard it as irrelevant to the decision which I have to take and I do not take it into account at all.'[1]

That might also apply to professional opinions about treatment that appear to be derived (or influenced by) the professional's personal religious view. Yet, it seems premature to exclude all religious values from consideration. We have noted several times that all decisions about life-sustaining treatment include values, and that many in society apply their own personal religious values to decisions about treatment for themselves. Nonreligious health professionals also apply values to determinations about the best interests of a child. It would seem unfair to allow nonreligious health professionals to include their values in an assessment of the reasonableness of treatment, while excluding those with religious beliefs.

Moreover, there might also be a concern that disallowing professionals from drawing on personal religious values in justifying an opinion about treatment would not change their view, but would lead them to conceal their religious views and just express their justification in terms of other more socially acceptable reasons or medical reasons. The hypothetical Jehovah's Witness haematologist might point to medical literature on the dangers of blood transfusion and on the possible benefits of nonblood alternatives (though at heart, their primary reason for reaching a particular point of view was not based on those factors). This is a positive in one way – it means that debate can focus on claims that are amenable to scientific and medical evidence. Those claims can be assessed and debated by others who do not share the haematologist's religious views. However, it also seems that this redirected justification is disingenuous.

We (the authors) disagree about the potential place of religious reasons in decisions about medical treatment for children. One of us (DW) is inclined to give them some weight, but the other (JS) believes, like Justice Holman, that they ought to be excluded from determinations about what is best for the child. The reason for this is that they are based on faith and are not revisable in the light of any evidence or argument. In this sense, they are unreasonable.[33]

For this book, we do not need to settle the question of whether professionals who are providing opinions about treatment should be allowed (or encouraged) to articulate their justification in terms of their personal religious beliefs. There are two possibilities. The first is that professionals are indeed encouraged to provide justifications in favour of treatment that others in society (who do not share their religious beliefs) are able to understand and accept. That would make it easier to assess whether their view about treatment is a reasonable one.

The second possibility is that professionals are encouraged to reflect on and articulate their personal religious or nonreligious values, and to cite them where they are relevant to their views on treatment. Some (religious or nonreligious) personal values would be able to be included as acceptable reasons in favour of treatment, while others would not. As noted earlier, only values that are incompatible with a general societal approach to decisions (such as a belief in the primacy of parental views about treatment, or a strong sanctity of life view) would be excluded as unreasonable.

Other religious values (for example, emphasising the value in the life of a disabled child) might still be included.

CONFLICT OF INTEREST

We have not included, in our description of characteristics that make a view reasonable or unreasonable, any mention of conflicts of interest. When there is disagreement between professionals, it is sometimes suggested that financial incentives could be motivating a view in favour of treatment. Privately funded treatment in some of these cases can be extremely expensive, and it could appear that specialists stand to gain financially from the treatment that they are offering. In the case of Charlie Gard, the Great Ormond Street team alleged that Professor Hirano retained a financial interest in some of the medicines that he was recommending for Charlie.[27]

However, such conflict claims are sometimes unfair. (Hirano denied that he had any financial interest in the medicines,[34] which were apparently relatively cheap to provide.) Moreover, they potentially apply not only to all private forms of medical treatment, but to most professional advice or services that we use in our everyday lives, including financial planning, house purchases, music lessons and travel agents. We don't think that our bank manager's mortgage advice automatically becomes unreasonable just because they or their bank will gain if we take up a mortgage. It would also be a mistake to assume that publicly funded specialists are automatically free from conflicts of interest. There could be powerful nonfinancial factors influencing opinions, including pride, prestige, academic reputation or promotion. For example, in the Jaymee Bowen case, private adult specialists accused public paediatricians of 'empire building'.[35]

Claims about conflict of interest where there is disagreement about medical treatment for a child sometimes appear dangerously *ad hominem*. (That term is the technical philosophical equivalent of 'playing the man, not the ball'.) In ethical debate, it is important to not attack the individual who is advancing an argument, but rather to address the argument itself. What we should be asking is whether there are clear, relevant reasons to support the view that someone is advancing. If there are, then it does not refute their view if they were to be paid to provide treatment. If there are not clear, relevant reasons, their view would be unreasonable even if they were offering their services for free.

Of course, it would be legitimate to ask anyone providing an expert opinion in a dispute to declare any interests in the treatment they are recommending. Transparency about interests is an important way to identify potential conflicts and to reduce their influence. However, we shouldn't dismiss opinions just because of a possible conflict. One way to neutralise such concerns would be to seek corroboration from other experts who do not have a financial stake in a decision.

To sum up the argument so far, we have suggested that, where there is reasonable disagreement about providing (or limiting) medical treatment for a child, we should, in general, allow parents to decide (we will return shortly to one limit to this). This accords with our suggestion in previous chapters that, where there is a possibility (based upon a reasonable evaluation of the facts) that treatment would be beneficial, it would be permissible for treatment to be provided or continued.

We have provided some considerations that might help to determine whether disagreement is reasonable or unreasonable:

Do those who are offering an opinion about treatment have knowledge of the relevant facts about the child's condition?

Do they have relevant expertise? Are they prepared (and able) to provide the treatment?

Can those offering treatment provide clear reasons in support of their view?

Does their opinion appear to be sensitive to changes in circumstance or evidence? Would they be willing to revise their view?

Is the opinion based on reasons that wider society has rejected as not relevant or unacceptable?

Limits to reasonable dissensus

Even if there is reasonable disagreement about whether treatment should be provided, there is another factor that may put a limit on whether treatment can be provided. That factor is the impact of providing treatment on other patients. Limited healthcare resources and scarcity may mean that treatment cannot be ethically provided – even if (thinking only about the interests of the patient) it would be reasonable to do so.

The next question, then, is how to determine where the boundaries are of reasonable disagreement – how to apply resource limits. We started to address that question in Chapter 4, suggesting that, where resources are scarce, it would be prudent to provide treatment that is probably of overall benefit and probably falls within the affordability limits of the health system. Yet, that does not solve the problem. There may be further disagreement about whether or not treatment will probably benefit the patient and whether or not it is affordable. It is highly likely that, within the medical profession and the wider community, there would be disagreement about how to evaluate the benefits of treatment (for example, whether or how to include considerations of quality of life) and where to set the threshold for judging treatment to be unaffordable.

We have endorsed a broadly pluralist approach to thinking about best interests and the benefits and burdens of treatment. However, we cannot apply a dissensus approach to decisions about provision of limited healthcare resources. To return to the analogy of dividing up a cake between a group of hungry people it would be as if we asked each person in turn to cut themselves what they feel would be a reasonable slice. People might be considerate of others and only take a small slice. Yet, some may decide that they should have a bigger piece, leaving the last members of the group with tiny slices or none at all. As another example, think about all the different priorities that face countries when they are dividing up the budget. There are a wide range of things that people might think are important to spend money on – education, health, infrastructure, culture, defence, foreign aid, etc. People may have very different priorities, and there would be a range of different reasonable ways of allocating the budget. However, if a country were to allocate money to just any priority or any budget item that could be judged reasonable by someone in society, it would quickly run out of funding.

When dividing a cake, or dividing up a country's budget, there is a responsibility to decide collectively (rather than individually) how to approach the task. In some cases, there may be an obvious fair solution that everyone could accept (e.g., dividing the cake equally so that everyone can have an identical slice). In more complex cases, it is necessary to decide between priorities or strategies. The standard approach to that problem is a democratic solution: resources are allocated based on the views of the majority.

When we are thinking about provision of scarce or limited healthcare resources, there is a need for consensus rather than dissensus. We cannot provide all treatment that could be judged reasonable to provide. Instead, we need to set boundaries for provision of treatment that are acceptable to most people within a society. We will make some more concrete proposals for how this might be approached in the next chapter; however, it is worth highlighting that reasonable pluralism is still relevant for resource allocation. When decision makers are deciding how to allocate resources, they need to be aware of the range of views within the community. They shouldn't just spend money on those resources that they would personally endorse or think are most important. For national budgets, it would be useful to know which areas are seen as priorities by different people, as well as the reasons underlying those views. A fair process of budget allocation should take those different priorities into account. In the same way, when it comes to medical treatment, it is important for those who are deciding to be aware of reasonable differences in opinion and to be prepared to accommodate those if possible.

As an example of how this might be applied, healthcare systems, whether they are public systems (like the NHS) or private insurance systems, will often look to scientific evidence to identify the best treatment for a given health condition. If those treatments provide sufficient benefit relative to their cost (if they fall below a cost-effectiveness threshold), they will be funded. However, in some cases, patients may have reasons to prefer alternative medical treatments. That might be because the alternative treatment avoids side effects or risks that are particularly important to an individual patient. (One example of this that we discussed in the previous chapter was the case of Ashya King.) Or it may be that some patients (or doctors) have different interpretations of the available evidence and disagree with the conventional view about what would be best. We have elsewhere argued that patients should be allowed to access reasonable suboptimal or alternative treatments that are cost-equivalent – i.e., they would not cost any more to the insurer or public health system than the standard treatment.[36] However, if we are serious about the importance of respecting different views within the community, societies should potentially also be willing to accommodate some alternative medical treatments that are not cost-equivalent, that are at least somewhat more expensive than the standard of care. When they should do this, and how much more expensive the treatment could be and still be provided, will potentially depend on the reasonableness of the request.[37]

This last point may be relevant to observed differences between different parts of the world in which treatments parents are allowed to choose for their child. We noted previously that some societies have made decisions that effectively exclude certain views about treatment as being unreasonable. Consideration of limited healthcare resources provides another reason that will influence the range of cases where parents are able to choose treatment. To put it bluntly, countries that are wealthier, countries where there is greater access to medical treatment, can afford to be more open-minded about providing treatment in cases of disagreement. The zone of parental discretion (which we described in Chapter 6) will be wider in societies that have more intensive care beds and more ability to accommodate parental requests for treatment without thereby harming other children. Fig. 7.1 illustrates three different hypothetical countries and the influence of resources on the zone of parental discretion:

Country A is a moderately well-resourced country like the UK. If the benefit of treatment (relative to cost/burden) is sufficiently high, treatment will be provided even if parents refuse consent. If the benefit is low, treatment will not be provided even if parents desire it.

Country B is a country with little resource limits on healthcare (for example, Sweden). The zone of discretion is shifted downward (there is less scope for parents to refuse treatment). There may be an expanded zone of parental discretion, allowing treatments even where the benefit is very low, and parents' desire for treatment may be overruled rarely.

Country C is a hypothetical low-resource country (for example, India). The zone of discretion is shifted upwards – some treatment may not be able to be provided even if potentially beneficial. There may be greater scope for parents to refuse treatment because they are self-funding treatment and there is little scope for the state to pay for treatment and ongoing care for a child.

Conclusion

To sum up, we have outlined in this chapter the relevance of disagreement for decisions about treatment. Where there is disagreement, and where that disagreement appears to be reasonable (e.g., in knowledge of relevant facts, apparently open to revision, based on acceptable values), it would be permissible to either provide or to withhold treatment. Reasonable dissensus helps to set out the range of treatment options that could possibly be respected. However, since decisions to provide treatment may also impact on others, in addition we need to seek reasonable consensus about how to allocate our limited healthcare resources. That consensus should be based on an appreciation of the range and reasonableness of views about treatment.

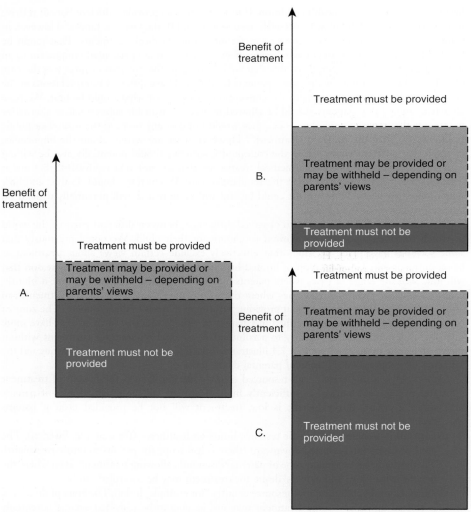

Fig. 7.1 The zone of parental discretion about treatment and three different hypothetical countries (A: moderately well-resourced, B: well-resourced, C: low-resource). The zone where parents may decide about treatment is indicated on the chart as 'light green'.

That may seem all well and good in theory – but how would it actually be applied? In the next chapter, we will look to develop a practical framework for deliberating on cases of disagreement about treatment.

References

1. An NHS Trust v MB [2006] *2 F.L.R. 319*.
2. Australian and New Zealand Intensive Care Society. (2003). '*Statement on withholding and withdrawing treatment Version 1.*' accessed 21/06/13 from <http://www.anzics.com.au/downloads/doc_download/136-the-anzics-statement-on-withholding-and-withdrawing-treatment-version-1>.

3. Intensive Care Society. (2003). *'Limitation of treatment on ICU.'* accessed 21/6/2013 from <http://www.ics.ac.uk/EasysiteWeb/getresource.axd?AssetID=469&type=full&servicetype=Attachment>.

4. General Medical Council (2010) *Treatment and care towards the end of life: good practice in decision making.* London, GMC.

5. Oxford English Dictionary (2013) *"consensus, n.".* Oxford University Press.

6. NSW Department of Health. (2005). *'Guidelines for end of life care and decision-making.'* accessed 19/7/2011 from <http://www0.health.nsw.gov.au/policies/gl/2005/GL2005_057.html>.

7. Baker, D. J. & Horder, J. (2013) *The sanctity of life and the criminal law : the legacy of Glanville Williams.* Cambridge, Cambridge University Press.

8. Dworkin, R. (1993) *Life's dominion : an argument about abortion and euthanasia.* London, HarperCollins.

9. Meyer, E. C., Ritholz, M. D., Burns, J. P. & Truog, R. D. (2006) Improving the quality of end-of-life care in the pediatric intensive care unit: parents' priorities and recommendations. *Pediatrics*, 117, 649-57.

10. Meert, K. L., Eggly, S., Pollack, M., Anand, K. J., Zimmerman, J., Carcillo, J., et al. (2008) Parents' perspectives on physician-parent communication near the time of a child's death in the pediatric intensive care unit. *Pediatr Crit Care Med*, 9, 2-7.

11. Melia, K. M. (2001) Ethical issues and the importance of consensus for the intensive care team. *Soc Sci Med*, 53, 707-19.

12. Meisel, A., Snyder, L. & Quill, T. (2000) Seven legal barriers to end-of-life care: myths, realities, and grains of truth. *JAMA*, 284, 2495-501.

13. Frost, D. W., Cook, D. J., Heyland, D. K. & Fowler, R. A. (2011) Patient and healthcare professional factors influencing end-of-life decision-making during critical illness: a systematic review. *Crit Care Med*, 39, 1174-89.

14. Wilkinson, D. J. & Truog, R. D. (2013) The luck of the draw: physician-related variability in end-of-life decision-making in intensive care. *Intensive Care Med*, 39, 1128-32.

15. Lofmark, R., Nilstun, T., Cartwright, C., Fischer, S., van der Heide, A., Mortier, F., et al. (2008) Physicians' experiences with end-of-life decision-making: survey in 6 European countries and Australia. *BMC Med*, 6, 4.

16. Gramelspacher, G. P., Zhou, X. H., Hanna, M. P. & Tierney, W. M. (1997) Preferences of physicians and their patients for end-of-life care. *J Gen Intern Med*, 12, 346-51.

17. Sprung, C. L., Carmel, S., Sjokvist, P., Baras, M., Cohen, S. L., Maia, P., et al. (2007b) Attitudes of European physicians, nurses, patients, and families regarding end-of-life decisions: the ETHICATT study. *Intensive Care Med*, 33, 104-10.

18. Gipson, J., Kahane, G. & Savulescu, J. (2014) Attitudes of lay people to withdrawal of treatment in brain damaged patients. *Neuroethics*, 7, 1-9.

19. Sprung, C. L., Maia, P., Bulow, H. H., Ricou, B., Armaganidis, A., Baras, M., et al. (2007a) The importance of religious affiliation and culture on end-of-life decisions in European intensive care units. *Intensive Care Med*, 33, 1732-9.

20. Schneiderman, L. J., Kaplan, R. M., Rosenberg, E. & Teetzel, H. (1997) Do physicians' own preferences for life-sustaining treatment influence their perceptions of patients' preferences? A second look. *Camb Q Healthc Ethics*, 6, 131-7.

21. Barnato, A. E., Hsu, H. E., Bryce, C. L., Lave, J. R., Emlet, L. L., Angus, D. C., et al. (2008) Using simulation to isolate physician variation in intensive care unit admission decision making for critically ill elders with end-stage cancer: a pilot feasibility study. *Crit Care Med*, 36, 3156-63.

22. Wilkinson, D., Truog, R. & Savulescu, J. (2016) In favour of medical dissensus: why we should agree to disagree about end-of-life decisions. *Bioethics*, 30, 109-18.

23. Wilkinson, D. (2017) Conscientious Non-objection in Intensive Care. *Camb Q Healthc Ethics*, 26, 132-142.

24. Janis, I. L. (1982) *Groupthink : psychological studies of policy decisions and fiascoes.* Boston, Houghton Mifflin.

25. McLean, S. A. (2007) What and who are clinical ethics committees for? *J Med Ethics*, 33, 497-500.

26. Berlin, I. (1998) On pluralism. *New York review of books.* New York. Accessed from <https://www.cs.utexas.edu/users/vl/notes/berlin.html>.

27. Great Ormond Street Hospital for Children. (2017). *'GOSH's position statement hearing on 24 July 2017.'* accessed 27 July from <http://www.gosh.nhs.uk/news/latest-press-releases/gosh-position-statement-issued-high-court-24-july-2017>.

28. Great Ormond St v Yates & Ors [2017] *EWHC 1909 (Fam)* (24 July 2017).

29. Great Ormond Street Hospital v Yates & Ors [2017] *EWHC 972 (Fam)* (11 April 2017).

30. D, Re (Medical Treatment) [2017] *EWCOP 15* (05 September 2017).
31. JS (Disposal of Body), Re [2016] *EWHC 2859 (Fam)* (10 November 2016).
32. Barilan, Y. M. (2015) Rethinking the withholding/withdrawing distinction: the cultural construction of "life-support" and the framing of end-of-life decisions. *Multidiscip Respir Med*, 10, 10.
33. Savulescu, J. (1998) Two worlds apart: religion and ethics. *J Med Ethics* 24 (6):382-4.
34. Bosely, S. (2017) US doctor's intervention in Charlie Gard case 'raises ethical questions'. *The Guardian*. Accessed from <https://www.theguardian.com/uk-news/2017/jul/25/michio-hirano-us-doctor-intervention-charlie-gard-case-raises-ethical-questions>.
35. Laurance, J. (1998) Child B: the truth about her last days. *Independent*. Accessed from <http://www.independent.co.uk/life-style/child-b-the-truth-about-her-last-days-1159951.html>.
36. Wilkinson, D. & Savulescu, J. (2017) Cost-equivalence and pluralism in publicly-funded health-care systems. *Health Care Anal*.
37. Nair, T., Savulescu, J., Everett, J., Tonkens, R. & Wilkinson, D. (2017) Settling for second best: when should doctors agree to parental demands for suboptimal medical treatment? *J Med Ethics*, 43:831-840.

CHAPTER 8

Embracing disagreement

'"Consider your verdict," the King said to the jury.
"Not yet, not yet!" the Rabbit hastily interrupted.
"There's a great deal to come before that!"'

Alice's Adventures in Wonderland, Lewis Carroll

So far in this book, we have explored some of the reasons that disagreement can be so intractable in cases like the Charlie Gard case: decisions turn on questions of value for which there is not an obvious correct answer. Our increasingly diverse and pluralistic societies comprise people from a range of social, cultural and religious backgrounds who are going to bring very different values to questions about quality of life and mortality. In addition, there are particular challenges relating to medical science and medical knowledge in the 21st century that actually make disagreement more likely. Scientific advances mean that the evidence base for prognosis and for medical treatments is complex, contested and constantly changing. Sometimes people hope that these technical improvements will make decisions in the future easier. Yet, genomic information may, paradoxically, actually create greater uncertainty. There may be extremely limited or no evidence that relates to the current patient. Evidence of a specific genetic profile can also call into question whether evidence relating to other patients should be extrapolated to the current patient. Moreover, there is a shifting medical information dynamic; because of the internet, patients and families have access to a huge amount of medical and scientific information. This information can be empowering – it alerted Connie Gard to a possibility for her son. It can give families access to new and evolving treatments that have not yet reached mainstream medicine. However, this information can also sometimes be misleading. It can feed into mistrust of health professionals and contribute to families feeling that they must battle with doctors to obtain what would be best for their loved one.

In the previous chapter, we started to outline how disagreement might be incorporated into a framework for decisions. Reasonable disagreement or dissensus can be used to identify a range of options that could be ethically permissible. We still need, though, to seek agreement or consensus about where and how to allocate resources. The aim in this chapter is to propose some more concrete solutions that could help healthcare systems to navigate, negotiate and resolve future disputes. Whilst we do not claim that these proposals are the only ways for societies to resolve medical treatment disputes, they provide definite advantages over the status quo, and thus merit serious consideration.

Nonsolutions and solutions

Previous chapters have identified some of ways that healthcare systems currently attempt (and fail) to deal with disagreement. We will identify these here; each will point to a separate element of the solutions that are needed.

  1. Exclusive focus on the interests of the child

As described in Chapters 2, 3 and 4, existing processes for dealing with disagreements about medical treatment usually focus on the question of whether treatment would be in the best interests of the child (or would harm the child). They ignore the issue of whether treatment is affordable, or whether, given its scarcity, provision of treatment to one patient would potentially harm other patients. They ignore questions of distributive justice. This exclusive focus is a mistake, as the problem of limited resources is a genuine and relevant ethical consideration. It may be more significant in less well-resourced publicly funded healthcare systems; however, it is a potential consideration for scarce treatment in all healthcare systems. Failure to distinguish these separate reasons to limit treatment can lead to two different serious problems. It can mean that possibly beneficial treatment in intensive care (or other areas of the hospital) is provided or continued for a long period of time, even though it is unaffordable or likely denies treatment to other patients.

Alternatively, conflation of the two separate ethical justifications means that possibly beneficial treatment is not provided, yet patients are unaware that this is because of limited healthcare resources. That denies patients or families the opportunity to petition governments, insurers or other doctors for greater investment of resources. It also may mean that they are denied the opportunity to seek separate (philanthropic or private) funding for treatment.

This is not to deny that in some cases the two reasons will converge. It may be the case that treatment should not be provided because it would both be harmful to the patient and an unjust use of limited resources. It will also often be the case that treatment should be provided because it would be both of benefit to the patient and a reasonable use of limited resources to do so. However, the reasons will sometimes also come apart. We need to have separate thresholds for these different decisions – the level at which treatment cannot be provided because of scarcity/cost, and the level at which treatment should not be provided because of harm. We will need different frameworks and may need a different way of reaching those different decisions.

2. Attempting to derive substantive criteria for nonprovision of treatment

Next, there has often been a temptation to try to define when treatment should be regarded as being futile (or, conversely, when it would be medically indicated). As we discussed in Chapter 2, this search has, ironically, itself often been futile because of the difficulty in both identifying clear criteria for futility, as well as in determining whether or not they apply in a particular case.

This problem potentially also applies to criteria for provision (or nonprovision) of treatment on the basis of limited resources. There again, there is considerable uncertainty and disagreement about where to draw thresholds for provision of treatment, how to assess different factors that might be included in thresholds (for example, how to or whether to assess quality of life) and whether or not thresholds are met for individual patients. The problem of uncertainty and disagreement is perhaps less intractable for resource questions than the problem of defining futility. That is partly because comparisons between patients (like the question of who is taller) are sometimes easier than evaluations for an individual patient (Is she tall?). Public healthcare systems or insurers also have to draw the line somewhere. They have no choice but to make decisions to provide some treatments and to not provide others. There will always be some degree of arbitrariness about such decisions; that is unavoidable.

Because of the difficulty in defining medical futility, there has been a move away from substantive criteria towards identifying a fair process for deciding whether or not treatment would be futile.[1,2] Following point #1, we need a fair process for deciding separately whether treatment would be unaffordable/unfair to provide, and whether it must not be provided (out of concern for the interests of the patient). We need to supplement this fair process with the development of general criteria for provision of treatment that could give families, clinicians and the community some guidance in situations where treatment is either likely or unlikely to be provided.

3. Reliance on the courts to make difficult ethical decisions

In many jurisdictions, if parents and health professionals cannot agree about treatment for a child, the only option is to go to court. In Chapter 1, when we described the series of legal hearings and appeals in the Charlie Gard case, it will have been clear that there are very significant downsides to relying on the courts to resolve treatment disputes. Legal processes are costly for the health system and for families (in the absence of legal aid funding or pro bono support). They can be lengthy and lead to long delays in decisions. As noted in Chapter 1, the Gard case involved five different court judgments at four separate levels of the court. It took 5 months from the hospital's initial application to the court until the final sad conclusion. Whatever our view about the case, that delay appears deeply regrettable. For those who agree with Charlie's parents that he should have had a chance to receive the nucleoside therapy, the long drawn out court process meant that he missed any opportunity to benefit. For those who regard continued intensive care as not in Charlie's interests, the court process and series of appeals meant that he received 5 months of potentially unpleasant treatment without benefit. For those who are concerned about the use of scarce intensive care resources, the court process meant that an intensive care bed was unavailable for another patient for 5 months. The average length of stay for children in paediatric intensive care is about 6.5 days in the UK.[3] On average then, a paediatric intensive care bed would be used by 22 children over a 5-month period. Court processes are also, by their nature, often adversarial, taking a considerable emotional toll on families and healthcare staff. The adversarial approach may entrench existing conflict, while making compromise or agreement more difficult. Although it may be possible to protect the identity of those involved, sometimes the consequence of the legal process is that personal medical details and family dynamics, as well as deeply private and tragic ethical decisions, are made public. In the Gard case, the public attention that accompanied the court case led to both his parents and the health professionals involved receiving hate mail.

It may be that, in some cases, court involvement is unavoidable. We might paraphrase Winston Churchill's sentiment about democracy: no one pretends that the courts are perfect or all-wise. They may be the worst place to make decisions, except for all the other alternatives.

However, perhaps it is premature to rule out all the other alternatives? There may be ways to avoid disagreements about treatment from becoming intractable. There may be alternative venues for dispute resolution. We will argue, in particular, that decisions about resource allocation should not be made by the courts.

Avoiding disagreement?

Before looking at ways to resolve disagreements, it is important to consider whether there are ways to avoid disagreements or to reduce the chance of them escalating into more serious disputes about treatment.

COMMUNICATION

There are few research studies that have ever formally evaluated ways to reduce conflict in end-of-life decisions.[4] One option that appears attractive, at least in theory, would be to focus on the training of health professionals. Many patient complaints relate to issues around communication.[5] Although it has not been proven to reduce disagreement, it seems highly likely that more or better training in communication might help professionals in their interactions with families around challenging treatment decisions.[6] Better skills in listening to patients and families and identifying and responding to their concerns might help to avoid misunderstanding or resentment. Improved ability to sensitively convey information about a patient's medical condition might help families to understand what is at stake and why professionals feel that a particular option would not be helpful. When families feel that they are being listened to and can understand a patient's medical situation, it seems likely that they would maintain trust in the professionals and be less inclined to seek alternative views or treatments.

Better communication is likely to be helpful. Indeed, it is hard to see any downside to improving communication skills – apart, perhaps, from the need for professionals to devote more time to interactions with families. However, it is not necessarily going to prevent all disagreements – partly because of the value differences that sometimes lead families and healthcare teams to different views about treatment. One qualitative study of disagreement in an adult intensive care unit in Belgium highlighted the very different perspectives of family and staff.[7] Both groups were focused on doing the best for the patient and on providing good care, yet this meant very different things to different groups. For the healthcare team, 'good care' was understood through a biomedical lens, in terms of somatic pathology, biological processes and medical diagnoses and treatments. By contrast, the families were reported to understand 'good care' in a more holistic way that included psychological, social and religious factors. The researchers identified ethnocultural differences between families and professionals as contributing to and reinforcing conflict.

So, in addition to skills in communication, health professionals, particularly those who work in the high stakes intensive care environment, need skills and training in ethics.

The purpose of ethics education here is not (merely) to tell professionals about ethical rules, concepts or principles. Instead, doctors and other health professionals need to be skilled in identifying and understanding the difference between facts and values, as well as the nature of value disagreements. Recognising disagreements that are based on different values is important because it suggests that some solutions will not work. Faced with family members who have a different view about treatment, clinicians are sometimes tempted to seek out more medical test results, further scientific evidence or more expert opinions that support their view about a patient's diagnosis or prognosis. Yet, where the underlying issue is value disagreement rather than factual disagreement, that evidence or those opinions may not be relevant, and may have no impact at all on a family's views about treatment. Professionals also need to appreciate the influence of values on their own views about treatment. It is important for them to be aware of the range of different reasonable perspectives on treatment amongst other health professionals and within the wider community. It is vital that professionals reflect and understand that patients and families will make decisions that differ from the decisions that the professional would make for themselves and their own family. They should be prepared to be tolerant of and to support decisions that they do not personally endorse.[8]

MEDIATION

Whereas education about ethics and communication might help reduce future cases of disagreement, that is not going to be helpful where disagreement has already occurred. It may be possible, at least in some cases, to reopen lines of communication that have closed and to help avoid further escalation of disagreement. In the Gard case, the judge mentioned the potential for some form of mediation or facilitation to avoid the need to resort to the court. Mediation has been proposed as a way to respond to apparently intractable disputes around treatment for children.[9] It involves a neutral external facilitator who is tasked to help parties to reach a negotiated resolution that they can both accept. The mediator does not take sides and does not make a decision. As an example, in the setting of medical negligence claims, a pilot mediation scheme helped identify the underlying causes of disagreement and rebuild relationships.[10]

Formal mediation uses trained external facilitators in established cases of conflict. There may also be value in teaching health professionals mediation skills that could be used informally at an earlier stage. After introduction of a pilot training program in a UK children's hospital, staff reported changes in their practice, including having a greater ability to recognise conflicts that were developing and feeling better able to manage and deescalate conflict.[11]

Side-stepping disagreement (avoiding unnecessary agreement)

The measures described previously may have an important role to play in helping reduce cases of disagreement or helping reach agreement in situations of established conflict. Yet, there is one group of situations where there is no need to seek agreement. Indeed, it would be arguably wrong to do so.

We suggested that there needs to be clear separation of situations where treatment is not being provided because of resource limitations. One reason for doing this is because in those situations it would be unfair to ask patients or families to agree with a decision not to provide treatment.

For example, imagine a situation where an organ has become available that would help two patients on the waiting list for a liver transplant, Carl and Adam. Both would benefit from the transplant (imagine too that they have been waiting for a similar period of time). However, Carl is now gravely ill and will almost certainly die without the transplant. Adam is much more stable, and there is a reasonable chance that another organ will become available for him. Some people might be tempted to toss a coin to decide who should get the liver. However, most people, we suspect, would agree with us that doctors should give the liver to Carl because of his more urgent medical need. If that is right, it would be wrong to ask Adam to give up his chance at the liver. That is for two reasons – if Adam refused, and his wish were respected, we would then be making an unfair decision, allowing Carl to die by giving Adam the liver. Alternatively, if doctors overruled Adam's refusal, giving the organ to Carl anyway, it would seem absurd and unfair to have asked Adam in the first place. There is no point asking someone to decide, if their choice is going to be ignored.

In a similar way, if the reason not to provide or continue life-sustaining treatment in intensive care is because of resource scarcity, it would be unfair to ask families to agree to this decision. Mediation may be beside the point.

The important question, then, is how to decide when agreement or consent is unnecessary – when treatment should not be provided because of scarcity.

POLICY

One approach to answering that question is to make such decisions at the level of policy. Health systems should formally evaluate treatments – for example, based on evidence of cost-effectiveness – and decide for the population whether or not treatment is provided. The National Institute for Health and Care Excellence (NICE) in the UK regularly makes these sorts of determinations about whether or not to make particular treatments available within the NHS. Health insurers also routinely make decisions about coverage – whether certain treatments will be reimbursed within particular plans. There are also professional guidelines or policy statements that set out 'indications' or 'contraindications' for treatment, identifying whether and when treatment will be provided.

These policy-level approaches to treatment are important, and should continue. They are, however, not enough. They do not solve the problem of allocating scarce resources, for several reasons. First, scarce treatments like extracorporeal membrane oxygenation (ECMO), intensive care or transplantation of solid organs, simply cannot be provided to all who could potentially benefit. There is a need to decide who will be treated, and policy makers are not always able (or willing) to do that. Second, whilst treatments may be cost-effective across a population or across large patient groups, they are not always uniformly cost-effective: there may be some patients for whom treatment would be much more costly or much less effective. Again, policy could make those distinctions, but often it does not. Third, policy-level decisions are often unhelpful in contested cases. This can be, for example, because the treatment is novel and has not yet been formally evaluated; because the patient's condition is rare, and policy evaluations (for other patients) are not relevant; or because the evidence that was previously assessed is now out of date. We have noted already that scientific and medical advances make it even more challenging to define medically futile treatment. The move to precision or genomic medicine will create smaller and smaller classes of patients. It will be difficult to extrapolate from blunt large group data to finely characterised small groups.

BEDSIDE

The opposite approach to allocating scarce resources would be to make decisions at the bedside. Doctors would be asked to make 'clinical' decisions about whether, for example, to provide intensive care, offer surgery or list a patient for transplantation. Bedside rationing at some level is probably inevitable.[12] At present, in fact, it seems to be the main locus for allocating treatments like intensive care. Intensive care doctors take into account the availability of beds (as well as potential demand by other patients) when they are deciding whether to admit a patient to intensive care or to start a treatment like ECMO. However, this sort of bedside rationing also appears to be problematic for several serious reasons. Firstly, these decisions are often based on intuition, not high-quality evidence. Secondly, these decisions are not simply 'clinical' decisions. They are value judgments about the relative benefit of treatment and the best way to allocate resources. Bedside allocation puts doctors in the very difficult position of being torn between what would be best for (and desired by) the patient, and what would be a reasonable use of resources. Thirdly, such allocation appears to lack key elements of a fair approach to resource allocation, as such determinations are usually not transparent, the ethical basis for them is not explicit and they are not open to appraisal or appeal.[13]

What is needed is a fair process for making decisions about providing treatment that is able to make timely, contemporaneous assessments in relation to specific patients, and is also fair, transparent and accountable. Most importantly, such decisions should be scientifically informed and based on clear ethical reasoning. Here is one proposal for what such a process might look like.[a] We are particularly considering what treatments a public health system should provide. We will discuss how it could be applied to private systems.

A bilevel process model for allocating scarce resources
LEVEL 1
Process for policy determinations

Ideally, medical treatments (both new and existing) should be evaluated at the level of a health system – for example, by a body such as NICE. Those determinations should take into account evidence about the cost of treatment, as well as its benefits. They also need to take account of, and incorporate, societal values that apply to the treatment. Deliberation and debate should include awareness of the range of views within the profession about the treatment. Policy makers should make clear the ethical basis for decisions, and those decisions should be able to be scrutinised and subject to revision or appeal if they are irrational or unreasonable. After assessment, treatment could be classified into three categories:

1. Available: Where there is clear evidence that treatment is effective and affordable across a population, it would be made uniformly available (at least where particular criteria for provision of treatment are met). Examples include antibiotics for sensitive bacterial infection.

---

[a]This is a development of proposals we made elsewhere.[14]

2. Unavailable: Where there is clear evidence that treatment is not effective or not affordable across a population, it would not be available for any patient. Examples include whole MRI body screening for presymptomatic disease. (Unavailable treatments could be purchased privately.)

3. Provisional: Where treatment may not be consistently effective and affordable (including cases where there is a lack of evidence) or where treatment cannot be made uniformly available (because of scarcity), it could be made available conditionally or provisionally. Further assessment for individual patients would be needed. Novel or emerging treatments (depending on their cost) might be included in this category as a default. Treatments that are highly expensive and close to the cost-effectiveness threshold could also be provided provisionally. Because of potential scarcity, most of the life-saving treatments discussed in this book (intensive care, renal dialysis, organ transplantation, long-term ventilation) would fall into this category. Where treatment falls into the provisional category, there will be a need for a further stage or level of decision-making (see later). Policy makers should set out the types of general considerations that would need to be taken into account in individual cases. We will give examples of these in the following section.

LEVEL 2

Process for evaluating provisionally available treatment

For treatment that might or might not be reasonable to provide, depending on the circumstances, there would need to be a process for assessing whether it should be provided for an individual patient. We need a process that is responsive to the circumstances of an individual patient, but more robust than bedside rationing. It should be independent from those caring for the patient, to avoid perceived or real conflicts of interest. It needs clinical information, but also ethical evaluation and reflection.

For example, an independent panel that included medical experts, ethicists and patient or lay representatives could evaluate the specific details of a patient's clinical condition and review the reasons why intensive care treatment is judged to be reasonable to provide. The patient's consultant could make the case for treatment on behalf of the patient, but the patient or family might also be able to express their views about treatment. Independent opinions would be useful where the family or patient is seeking treatment that is not endorsed by the current clinical team. There are two different ways that this second level assessment might occur:

1. Prior assessment: Where treatment decisions do not need to be made urgently, the panel could be asked to make a decision before starting treatment.

2. Post hoc assessment (and time-limited trial): For treatment that must be provided urgently, if it is to be provided at all, it would not be possible for panels to assess and decide in advance whether treatment should be provided. However, treatment could, at least in some cases, be commenced and then reviewed. This would apply, for example, to intensive care admission. In that case, one option would be to provide a time-limited trial of treatment. At the end of the trial period, the panel could be asked to decide whether a further period of treatment should be provided. Formal review by the review panel may not be necessary in all cases (e.g., where the patient is obviously improving and unlikely to need much more time on respiratory support).[b]

---

[b]Post hoc review and trials of treatment would not be an option for some treatments, e.g., those involving urgent surgery or organ transplantation. These would need to be decided in a different way.

Critical Care Triage and Treatment Review Panel

We envisage that a specialised panel could review intensive care decisions (perhaps within a region). The model that we have in mind has some similarity with an existing model within the UK for considering requests for treatment. Within the NHS, Individual Funding Request (IFR) panels are available to assess requests for treatment that is not routinely available.[15] These panels comprise independent clinicians (including GPs) who assess evidence presented by the patient's own doctor on the effectiveness and cost-effectiveness of the treatment and the patient's clinical need, as well as the exceptional nature of a patient's request for that treatment.

However, what we are proposing differs from existing IFR panels in several ways. IFR panels only make decisions about treatment that is nonfunded. They therefore ask for evidence that a patient's situation is exceptional (in order to justify funding where it is not normally available). The model that we are describing explicitly accepts that treatment may be reasonable to provide for some patients – that is why treatment is classified as provisionally available. Evidence might be presented that the patient's condition is usual or nonexceptional. Second, we have implied that this treatment panel should have specific expertise in critical care. (We could imagine, for example, separate triage and treatment review panels for organ transplantation, home ventilation or other scarce treatment.) That would mean that at least some on the panel have relevant clinical expertise to assess the specific medical evidence relevant to a decision about treatment.

The membership of such panels should not be confined to health professionals. Although decisions about allocation of resources often depend on assessment of medical or scientific evidence, they are also fundamentally linked to ethical and value questions. The panel should engage in ethical deliberation and reasoning, and make the reasons for their decisions clear. Some members of the panel should have knowledge of the relevant ethical concepts, like distributive justice. Third, we have proposed that treatment review be combined with time-limited trials of treatment. This is necessary in the critical care context (or other contexts where care is ongoing) because, as noted, there would often be no possibility of prior assessment of treatment. (Prior assessment might be possible in situations where there is a question about whether patients with severe underlying morbidity should be admitted to intensive care in the event of deterioration. However, even in such cases, the answer may depend on whether the deterioration is acute and reversible, or progressive and irreversible.) Setting a specific time limit for a trial of treatment would allow evidence about the patient's clinical situation and their response to intensive care to be gathered and presented. It may also help to frame the nature of decisions in a way that is more socially acceptable. The default assumption in a time-limited trial of treatment is that, after a given period, treatment would be stopped. The Critical Care Triage and Treatment Review Panel (CTRP) proposed here would then be making a decision about continuing treatment or embarking on a further (time-limited) trial of treatment. This may be significant in one way: whilst there is ethical and legal consensus that there is no difference between withholding and withdrawing treatment, many professionals and others within the community find stopping treatment much more difficult.[16] It is sometimes suggested that patients acquire a right or a stronger claim to treatment once it has been started.[17] However, that claim would appear to be diminished or avoided if it is clear from the start that treatment is only being provided for a trial period. A CTRP would also separate considerations of the particular patients from broader distributive justice considerations, relieving the treating clinician from managing this tension with families.

At the policy level, decisions should be made about when treatment would be made available provisionally, but also whether it would be appropriate to review prospectively or after a trial of treatment. Policies should set out the duration of time-limited trials, as well as the general criteria that should be assessed to decide whether further treatment would be provided.

How long should trials be? That will partly depend on how long it would take to assess whether a patient is responding to treatment. It will depend on how long it would take to assemble the

CTRP and to reach a decision about further treatment. It will also depend on the scarcity or cost of the treatment. Where treatment is less scarce or more likely to be cost-effective, it may be reasonable to provide a longer treatment trial.

One practical option for intensive care units would be to base the duration of treatment trials on the timing of a common clinical decision point. When patients appear likely to require longer periods of support from breathing machines, doctors often decide to perform a procedure (tracheostomy) that moves the patient's breathing tube from their mouth (or nose) to the bottom of their neck. In adult intensive care, tracheostomy is often considered after patients have been ventilated for 4 to 7 days (and sometimes earlier[c]),[18] whereas this is typically undertaken much later in paediatric intensive care (often only after 2 weeks)[19] or neonatal intensive care (after 2–3 months, depending on the size of the baby).[20] It could be useful to explain to families that the patient is being provided with an initial trial period of orotracheal or nasotracheal respiratory support. Further ventilation (and tracheostomy) would only be considered if the CTRP judges that this would be reasonable (in the setting of scarce resources).[d]

Another clinical decision point is based on whether a patient would be eligible for long-term ventilation (e.g., home ventilation). Sometimes decisions about tracheostomies coincide with decisions about long-term ventilation (i.e., only patients who are candidates for long-term ventilation are offered tracheostomy). However, there is no theoretical reason why these could not be separated. Particularly where there is uncertainty about a patient's prognosis, it may be reasonable to perform a tracheostomy and embark on a further trial period of ventilator support, before then making a decision to move to a long-term ventilation program or to withdraw intensive care.

How would the review panel decide whether treatment should be provided (or continued)? As mentioned in the previous chapter, decisions to provide limited resources need to be made by agreement, and in line with wider social values. The CTRP decisions will be made by consensus rather than by dissensus. They should ideally be made on the basis of criteria or factors set out at the policy level. For example, in Chapter 4 we discussed how cost-effectiveness thresholds might be used to inform when it would be reasonable to provide intensive care – e.g., establishing a minimum chance of survival, duration of survival or maximum duration of treatment. The results of decisions by the CTRP could also be fed back into policy as a form of reflective equilibrium. For example, situations where treatment was always judged to be reasonable to provide might be used to set out criteria for provision of treatment (perhaps without need for CTRP review). Variation in decisions (in similar situations) would point to the need for clearer or more substantive policy guidance.

COST-EFFECTIVENESS-BASED THRESHOLD FOR PROVIDING SCARCE TREATMENT

Based on information about the usual costs and benefits of treatment, it would be possible to calculate some minimum conditions for cost-effective treatment. In Chapter 4, we gave the example that it would, in theory, be cost-effective to provide 20 days of intensive care to an adult with a more than 9% chance of survival (assuming full quality of life and survival for 10 years after intensive care). The CTRP could take a threshold like this and assess whether it is likely that a particular patient (who has received 10 days of intensive care) has a more than 9% chance of survival. Alternatively, they could undertake more complicated multifactorial modelling for an individual patient to assess the likelihood of treatment being cost-effective given a particular chance of survival, life expectancy, cost of treatment and/or quality of life. There is, of course,

[c]There is considerable debate about the merits of early or late tracheostomy in adult intensive care.
[d]There is no intrinsic moral significance of this time point. Tying assessment to the timing of tracheostomy is pragmatic and convenient rather than necessary. Treatment should be reviewed prior to tracheostomy, or post-tracheostomy wherever this is relevant.

likely to be uncertainty in any such assessment. Yet, this may still be useful as a reference point for debate and as a way to ensure that decisions are made consistently on the basis of factors judged to be relevant by wider society. Thresholds need to incorporate other social values, such as fairness. Wherever thresholds are set for provision of resources, the aim of the CTRP meeting would be to assess whether it is likely that treatment would be a fair use of limited resources (in which case treatment should be made available) or unlikely to be a fair use (in which case further treatment should not be provided from the public healthcare system). If there remains considerable uncertainty about whether treatment would represent a reasonable use of limited resources, it may be possible to embark on a further time-limited trial of treatment. Alternatively, it may be that patients are offered the option of accessing treatment outside the public healthcare system.

Example cost-effectiveness-based thresholds for providing expensive and intensive medical treatments[e]

1. Probability threshold: ECMO is potentially cost-effective for a newborn if their chance of survival is >1.4%
2. Duration threshold: Maximum duration of cost-effective ECMO (for a patient with a 25% chance of survival and a 20-year life expectancy): 13 days
3. Quality threshold: Minimum quality of life for performing a Fontan repair (assuming survival for 10 years): 0.1

Private healthcare systems

So far, we have focused on resource thresholds for publicly funded healthcare systems. It is worth recalling, though (see Chapter 4), that the same issues potentially apply to scarce treatment in privately funded systems. For example, US ethicists Norm Daniels and James Sabin have described the approach of some managed care organisations to deciding whether or not to fund experimental or innovative treatments.[23] Two organisations used a process of external expert review whenever patients sought last-chance therapies that the insurer's oncologists did not feel were beneficial. The independent panel conducted 'an expert clinical assessment of the potential value of the technology for a particular patient'. This appears similar to the IFR panels used in the NHS.

Intensive care units in privately funded healthcare systems could use a CTRP for evaluating whether intensive care could be provided or continued. Compared with public systems, there might be a longer trial period prior to review (if treatment is less scarce). CTRPs in the private sector might draw not on cost-effectiveness thresholds, but instead on other factors – for example, the level of demand and clinical need of other patients requiring intensive care, or just the cost of treatment. Where it appears likely that continuing intensive care would benefit the patient and not harm other patients (by denying them access to treatment), it would be reasonable to continue treatment. However, where it is unlikely that the benefit to the current patient would be significant and where treatment would harm other patients (by utilising a fixed resource), it would be reasonable not to provide further treatment in the intensive care unit.

DEMAND-BASED THRESHOLD FOR PROVIDING SCARCE TREATMENT

Where a healthcare system is unable to provide a treatment to all who could benefit from it (i.e., it is, by definition, 'scarce'), the hospital or treating team could audit the prognosis of patients

---

[e]For details and further discussion of how these are calculated.[21,22]

seeking treatment and the proportion of unmet demand. For example, a CTRP could assess the illness severity/chance of survival for patients referred for ECMO, as well as determining what proportion of referrals are declined. They might determine that 10% of patients referred are not able to be treated. They could then identify what approximate prognosis would correspond to the bottom tenth percentile at referral and use this as a guide to providing a trial of treatment. (If patients are treated who have a worse outlook than this, it is likely that other patients with higher chances would be denied treatment.) As noted in Chapter 4, to balance fairness with benefit, the CTRP could choose to deliberately lower the threshold to some degree – e.g., to the fifth percentile, accepting that this may reduce the overall numbers of children able to be saved, but giving some weight to fairness.

These thresholds could also be adjusted based on demand at a particular point in time. For example, if the ECMO centre currently has vacant beds, it might be possible to provide a trial of treatment even for a patient below the usual threshold. Conversely, seasonal high demand might lead to a temporary upward shift of the bar for treatment.

One additional advantage of this explicit process for allocating treatment is that gathering data about unmet demand (and the prognosis of patients excluded from treatment) could be used to make a case for seeking additional resources – e.g., more staff/equipment for intensive care/ECMO.

Embracing disagreement

We have argued that decisions to provide or not provide treatment on the basis of limited healthcare resources should be made by consensus, based on the values of a community. However, where there is disagreement between experts about the benefit or reasonableness of a treatment, or where there is disagreement between a family and health professionals, that may point to uncertainty about what the right thing to do is. In those circumstances, even if treatment is not able to be provided within a publicly funded healthcare system (or within a resource-limited private institution), it may still be ethical to provide it, for example, where treatment is privately funded, philanthropically funded or less scarce.

How should we decide whether or not to allow treatment in these circumstances? We suggested in the previous chapter that professional dissensus would provide evidence supporting reasonable disagreement about the benefits of treatment. The primary role of the CTRP that we have described earlier is to assess the reasonableness of providing treatment within a resource-limited healthcare system. However, it would make sense for them to separately consider the merits of the treatment if resources are not an issue.

Where treatment is proposed that is novel or unusual, it would be important to have experts who are offering the treatment give evidence directly to the panel. As noted in the previous chapter, where an expert is able to demonstrate that they are aware of the salient facts about the patient (e.g., they have reviewed the patient's condition in detail) and can articulate the reasons why they have reached their view about treatment, there would be a stronger case for that alternative being viewed as 'reasonable'. (Review in person might not always be feasible, where a second opinion is provided from overseas. A virtual second opinion, if systematic and thorough, might in some cases be sufficient.)[f] Fig. 8.1 indicates a schematic approach to a decision-making process. As suggested by the figure, where those who have reviewed treatment have had divided opinions about treatment, a family would be given the option of seeking alternative practitioners prepared to offer the treatment. The CTRP might also propose this option in situations where the panel

---

[f]A virtual second opinion that diverges from the opinion of those who have reviewed the patient would need to include review of the medical record and up-to-date clinical assessment, review of all test results, discussion of need for any further examination or test with clinicians via internet link and perhaps demonstration of any relevant bedside test or examination by internet link.

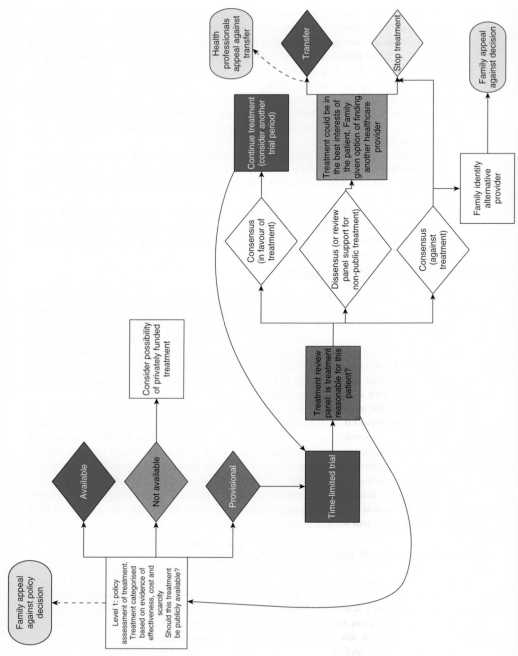

Fig. 8.1 A proposed approach to resolving disagreement about medical treatment for children

uniformly believes that treatment cannot be afforded within the public healthcare system, but at least some of the panel believe that it could nevertheless be in the child's best interests. In such circumstances, if a family has found a relevant health professional who is able and willing to provide the treatment, the presumption should be that they would be allowed to seek transfer of the child to the willing health professional's care.

Finally, if a CTRP has reviewed a child's situation, and there is no support for providing the treatment, the presumption would be that treatment would stop. In that situation, the absence of reasonable disagreement about the merits of treatment suggests that further treatment should not be provided.

We have suggested three possible points at which families might formally appeal against treatment decisions:

1. A family might appeal against the determination that treatment should not be available in the public healthcare system. As discussed in Chapter 4, courts will not usually over-rule decisions about provision of funding for treatment unless those decisions are clearly irrational. Courts have accepted that healthcare systems have finite resources and need to make difficult decisions. If a review panel has followed the correct process for assessing the merits of treatment (including, for example, listening to and taking account of different opinions), its decisions would normally stand. Where a court found that the process had not been adhered to, the decision would be referred back to the review panel.

2. Where treatment is not being publicly provided, but a family is proposing to transfer the child to another provider, it is possible that those currently treating the child would object to the transfer. They might, for example, regard the proposed treatment as harmful. For example, this could have been an option had our model been applied to the Jaymee Bowen case. The clinical team apparently felt that treatment was not in Jaymee's interests. The current treating team could appeal against the transfer on the basis of this concern about harm. However, we suggest that where the expert review panel is divided about the merits of treatment and there is a professional willing to provide the treatment, in most circumstances such an appeal would be unlikely to succeed.

3. We noted that where the treatment review panel all regard treatment as being unreasonable, such treatment would usually be withdrawn. In those circumstances, if a family were able to find another reasonable provider willing to provide treatment, that could either lead to a decision returning to the panel or a family could appeal directly to a court to allow transfer. As noted in the previous chapter, the court or review panel should review evidence of the reasonableness of the option. They might, for example, assess the reasons given for judging treatment to be beneficial and assess whether the view is reason-sensitive and the reasons given are acceptable and compatible with the values of wider society. The latter would be particularly important for proposed international transfer of a patient.

Advantages and disadvantages

The process that we have described in this chapter has the three features that we claimed were desirable in a system for addressing disagreements about treatment. First, it clearly separates decisions about allocating scarce and limited resources from decisions about the best interests of the patient. Second, we have tried to set out a fair process for reaching these two decisions. The resource decision could be reached at a policy level, though some treatments (particularly those that are scarce) will need further assessment at the level of the patient. We set out a process for reviewing provision of treatment that draws on medical expertise, but also includes ethical input. Third, this model avoids relying on the court for decisions. Most decisions, most of the time, would not require court input.

There are, however, possible concerns or objections to this new model.

IMPACT ON USUAL DECISION-MAKING

Decisions to limit life-sustaining treatment in intensive care occur on a daily basis. One immediate concern for clinicians might be that the model would create bureaucratic hurdles to those decisions, or might delay them, by requiring clinicians to seek out a treatment review panel. Yet, nothing in this chapter would impact on the decisions that doctors and families together make about life support. As we noted in the very first chapter, most such decisions are made by agreement. In cases of agreement, there would be no need to refer to the CTRP or to consider external opinions. In fact, there may be an advantage of the new model for those decisions made with families. By separating resource-based determinations from scarcity-based determinations, families may be reassured that the recommendations of the clinician are based purely on concern for the child's (or adult's) best interests. The model would reduce the need for bedside rationing in intensive care, allowing clinicians to focus on the patient in front of them.

ADDITIONAL LAYERS AND DELAYS PRIOR TO COURT

One concern might be that this model would not avoid cases of disagreement from reaching the court. The model allows families (or doctors) to appeal decisions, and so it might be thought to simply create extra unnecessary steps prior to legal review. However, as noted, we have envisioned a more limited role for courts in cases of disagreement. The court would be able to review the process of decision-making about provision of resources, but not the content. Where there are divided views about the benefit of treatment and a family has found an alternative professional prepared to provide it, the presumption would be in favour of allowing transfer of the patient. Where there is consensus within the CTRP that treatment would not be in the child's best interests, a family should only be able to appeal that decision if they are able to identify a professional who is willing and able to provide that treatment. (In the next section, we will compare the CTRP process with an existing US process for reviewing potentially futile medical treatment.)

INEQUALITY

The model that we have described separates the question of limited resources from the question of the best interests of the patient. It allows wealthy families to access treatment for a seriously ill child that is not available to families who are dependent on the public health system. That is likely to be distasteful to some (particularly those who are familiar with the egalitarian NHS). Serious inequalities in wealth are present in many societies. They are certainly unfair, and many people, including ourselves, feel that it would be much better if wealth were more equally distributed. However, it is also unfair to prevent families from paying for and accessing desired and potentially beneficial healthcare. As we have noted, public healthcare systems have real limits on the treatment that they are able to provide. Beyond those limits are some treatments that are potentially beneficial. We can reduce this problem by ensuring that our public healthcare systems are adequately funded and have enough intensive care beds, staff, etc. to provide most treatment that would be desirable and helpful. But if treatment is being denied because of limited resources, and if there is some reasonable basis for thinking that treatment would be of benefit, it would be wrong to prevent families from accessing treatment because of concern for equality. That would be a form of 'levelling down equality' that makes some people worse off, but no one better off.

ENCOURAGING CROWDSOURCING

In the Charlie Gard case, his family successfully raised a large sum of money to potentially fund his overseas medical treatment, which all agreed had very low chances of providing a relatively modest benefit. The model we have described might seem to encourage families to embark on this sort of fundraising. Yet, there are a range of ethical concerns about crowdsourcing for medical treatment.[24] For example, such campaigns appear to favour families with the skills to mount successful social media or conventional media campaigns, and their success may depend on attractive photos and heart-wrenching or unique stories (whereas those with equally serious but more commonplace or unattractive illnesses do not attract funds). They can compromise the privacy of children with chronic health conditions. It can be difficult for donors to know if needs are genuine, or how money would be used. Such crowdsourced funds can be misused and not used for the benefit of the child. Finally, there are concerns that such campaigns divert philanthropic donations from other causes that would be much more beneficial. (That is going to be of particular concern for the types of expensive and comparatively low benefit treatment that would be denied by treatment review panels.) For example, the money raised by the Gard's crowdsourcing campaign, if donated to an antimalaria charity, could have provided 640,000 bed nets to protect people living in regions affected by malaria from getting infected and potentially saved 533 lives.[25]

There are very important, pressing questions about how fundraising campaigns for healthcare should be organised, to protect both recipients and donors. There are also important ethical questions about where people should donate their money and whether they should always seek to do the most good with their donations. However, those questions are independent of questions about how to address disagreements between health professionals and families about treatment. (Issues about crowdsourcing apply even if there is no disagreement between doctors and parents, and also arise in health systems that do not make any explicit attempt to ration treatment.) We will have to set those questions aside for another day.

Comparison with existing models

The process that we have described for addressing disagreement about medical treatment has some similarities with existing models. This is a potential strength because it addresses potential concerns about feasibility.

We noted earlier that the treatment review panels we envisage have some similarities with IFR panels. That points to the acknowledged need to consider in individual cases whether treatment can be provided within a public healthcare system. It also suggests that (at least in the UK) it could be politically acceptable and possible to have a non–court-based process for decision-making about allocation of resources to specific patients. Of course, given the political sensitivity of 'rationing', that may be more challenging in other parts of the world, for example North America.

The CTRPs also have some similarities with a unique model developed and used in Texas over the last 2 decades for addressing futility disputes.[26] The Texas Advance Directives Act (TADA), which came into effect in 1999, includes a provision for resolution of treatment disputes. Where a family or patient is requesting life-sustaining medical treatment that the physician regards as inappropriate, the decision can be referred to a hospital ethics or medical committee. The committee hears evidence from health professionals and reaches a decision about the appropriateness of further treatment. Where the committee concludes that treatment is inappropriate, the hospital must make efforts to transfer the patient to another doctor prepared to provide the treatment, but if they are unable to do so within 10 days, the hospital may then withdraw treatment. There are limited avenues for legal appeal, and the health professionals and hospitals are legally protected if they follow the process set out in the Act.

The TADA model demonstrates that it is possible to have a nonjudicial process for reviewing medical treatment. A survey conducted by the Texas Hospitals Association in 2012 reported that TADA had been used 30 times by its 202 member hospitals between 2007 and 2012.[27] Of those cases, one-third of patients died during the process of reviewing treatment, whilst six patients were transferred to another hospital. Of the cases that reached that stage, the committee agreed with a decision to stop treatment in 7 out of 10 cases.

The CTRP that we have described also has some differences from the TADA process. These differences partly arise from the different role of treatment review that we have envisaged, but we have also sought to address some criticisms of TADA. First and foremost, the CTRP has an explicit role to consider issues of limited resources and whether it is reasonable to provide treatment within a public healthcare system. That may mean that there is more scope for transfer of patients than is possible in the Texan system (where decisions not to provide treatment are based on it being 'inappropriate'). Second, we have suggested that review panels should be independent from hospitals – they should not be hospital ethics committees (as occurs in Texas). This is to avoid conflict of interest, as well as a perception that decisions are being made by colleagues of treating doctors. Such panels could be set up regionally or nationally and draw on professionals (medical and nonmedical) from a range of institutions. Third, we have suggested that the CTRPs should base their decisions on criteria developed at a policy level. Furthermore, their decisions should be reviewed and used to feed back into further policy. Their reasoning should be publicly available and open to scrutiny, deliberation and debate. Fourth, by providing treatment 'provisionally' – for example, as a time-limited trial – the model reduces expectations of treatment continuing unabated and gives families a clear understanding up front that treatment will be reviewed after a period to assess whether further treatment would be of benefit.

Experimental treatment

We have described a general approach to disagreements about treatment, focussing on intensive care, because that has often been the site for disagreements. However, the model could be adapted to cases of experimental treatment. It could then be applied, for example, to situations where families are requesting innovative forms of anticancer treatment (as in the Ashya King case). Fig. 8.2 shows an adaptation of the model that we have described.

Policy determinations will often not have been conducted for experimental treatment. By definition, these are treatments that have not yet moved into standard care. They will usually not be able to be publicly funded (except perhaps as part of a clinical trial). If there is sufficient evidence of the costs and effectiveness of treatment, they should be assessed as usual (i.e., they could have the same sort of assessment that we described earlier). If there is no scientific evidence of the merits of a treatment (e.g., faith healing), it might be regarded in the same way as alternative medicines, i.e., that it will not be publicly funded, but might be sought privately. In situations where health professionals object to the treatment (e.g., because they believe it would be harmful to a child), they could refer the decision to a treatment review panel (or directly to a court).

If experimental treatment is available as part of a clinical trial, the ethics of treatment will be assessed by a research ethics committee. Treatment would usually be funded as part of the trial.

Where there is some evidence in favour of a treatment or some reason to believe that the intervention might have beneficial physiological effect (as in the case of nucleoside replacement), but the nature or degree of benefit is unclear and it is not available as part of a clinical trial, prior review by a treatment review panel would be necessary. (In situations of urgent need for treatment, a time-limited trial might be provided while organising review.) That is obviously exactly the situation that applied in the Gard case and in the case of Jaymee Bowen. The review panel in this case would primarily be assessing the benefits (and risks) of treatment (i.e., focused more on the best interests question than on the resources question). It might be composed of different members with different areas of expertise than the CTRPs described previously. If the panel decide strongly in favour of treatment, there would be a case for seeking a way to fund the treatment. That might be through a compassionate use scheme with the manufacturer, through funding set aside within a public health system specifically for innovative (perhaps last-ditch)

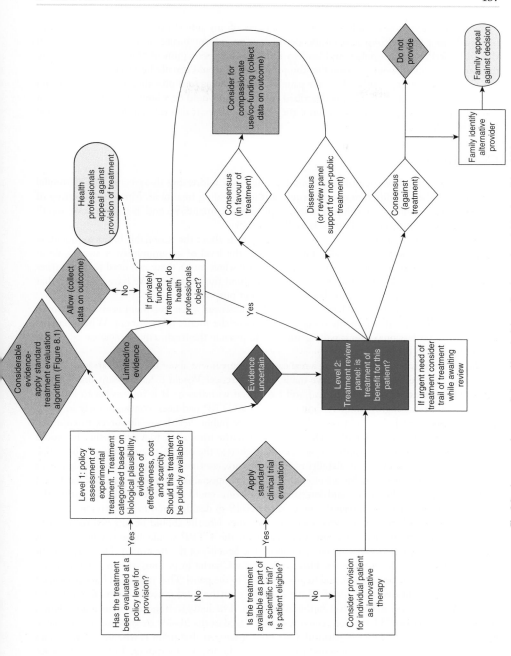

Fig. 8.2 A proposed approach to making decisions about experimental treatment for children.

therapies or through charitable funding. The effects of any intervention should be assessed as rigorously as possible from a scientific perspective to inform future decisions. That decision should be fed back into policy and lead to formal policy evaluation of this treatment. Where the panel is divided about the benefits, the presumption would usually be in favour of allowing self-funded treatment. Finally, where the panel is unanimous against providing treatment, it would usually not be provided, though, as described earlier, there would be a limited legal possibility of a family appealing against that decision if they have the support of a relevant health professional for their decision.

Conclusions

In this chapter, we have described a potential model for addressing disagreement. This model separates out the two different questions relevant to providing treatment. First, in the setting of scarcity or limited resources, is it reasonable to provide treatment? Second, is treatment of overall benefit to the patient (or would it be overall harmful)?

For the first question, there is a need to seek consensus about the reasonable limits to providing treatment. It may be possible to develop policies at the level of a community or society about those limits; however, for some treatments (particularly scarce ones), there will need to be a further assessment for individual patients about whether to fund the treatment. We have suggested that independent treatment review panels could serve that purpose.

For the second question, we have suggested that dissensus when treatment is reviewed would suggest the presence of reasonable disagreement about the merits of treatment. Where parents have a health professional who is willing and able to provide the treatment, in most cases parents should be able to do so.

We started this book by describing a real case of disagreement about medical treatment. Would the model that we have proposed have made any difference? Would it have meant that Charlie received treatment, or would treatment still have been withdrawn? It is impossible to know, in retrospect. It seems highly unlikely though, that, if a CTRP had been convened early in 2017, it would have been judged a reasonable use of scarce public healthcare resources to continue mechanical ventilation for Charlie. The chance of Charlie improving to a degree that he would be able to survive without a ventilator was remote, whereas the cost of treatment was substantial. Given the limitations on the availability of intensive care, continued treatment potentially meant that other children were unable to be admitted to the specialised intensive care unit at Great Ormond Street. Tracheostomy and long-term ventilation could not conceivably fall within the standard cost-effectiveness thresholds used in the NHS to decide when to fund treatment.

If the panel had then been asked to review whether Charlie should be allowed to travel to receive desired (self-funded) experimental treatment, the CTRP would have needed to assess whether there was reasonable disagreement about the benefits of the treatment. The panel might have asked the US expert Professor Hirano to review Charlie in person, or perhaps through a more detailed virtual consultation, and to give evidence to the panel. That might not have persuaded the panel if he appeared to be drawing on values (e.g., strong deference to parental autonomy) that are not acceptable in the UK. On the other hand, if he had given more convincing evidence, perhaps the panel would have been convinced that a trial of nucleoside therapy was a reasonable option, or at least not obviously harmful. One further issue at that point is whether there was an intensive care unit in the US prepared to accept Charlie for the treatment. In the final stages, there were units in both the US and Italy prepared to accept Charlie, but it is not clear what the situation was at the time of the first hearing. Given finite availability of intensive care beds, there should arguably also have been a CTRP at the proposed facility in the US. That panel might have looked at the demand for and availability of paediatric intensive care beds and assessed whether provision of a space for Charlie would have deprived other children of the opportunity for treatment. If that panel agreed to offer treatment, it might have specified a time-limited trial with set endpoints, for example improvement in EEG and in muscle power. In the absence of improvement, the expectation would be that treatment would be withdrawn.

We suggest that a different approach to disagreement about medical treatment might have made it possible to give fair attention to different views about Charlie's condition, while also setting necessary limits on treatment that can be provided and that can be demanded by parents. We hope, though we do not know, that this different approach might have led to a speedier, less painful, less public resolution of the dispute.

As a final illustration of the process, the next chapter tries to imagine what the outcome could be in a future case. It draws on a condition with some similarities to Charlie Gard's and a new cutting-edge experimental treatment of uncertain benefit.

References

1. Fine, R. L. & Mayo, T. W. (2003) Resolution of futility by due process: early experience with the Texas Advance Directives Act. *Ann Intern Med*, 138, 743–746.
2. Stewart, C. (2011) Futility Determination as a Process: Problems with Medical Sovereignty, Legal Issues and the Strengths and Weakness of the Procedural Approach. *J Bioeth Inq*, 8, 155–163.
3. Paediatric Intensive Care Audit Network. (2016). '*November 2016 Annual Report*.' from <https://www.hqip.org.uk/public/cms/253/625/19/680/PICANet%20Annual%20Report%202016.pdf?realName=ETGnJq.pdf&v=0>.
4. Hillman, K. & Chen, J. (2008). '*Conflict resolution in end of life treatment decisions: An Evidence Check rapid review brokered by the Sax Institute* (http://www.saxinstitute.org.au) for the Centre for Epidemiology and Research.' from <http://www.health.nsw.gov.au/research/Documents/14-conflict-resolution-end-of-life.pdf>.
5. Reader, T. W., Gillespie, A. & Roberts, J. (2014) Patient complaints in healthcare systems: a systematic review and coding taxonomy. *BMJ Qual Saf*, 23, 678–689.
6. Levin, T. T., Moreno, B., Silvester, W. & Kissane, D. W. (2010) End-of-life communication in the intensive care unit. *Gen Hosp Psychiatry*, 32, 433–442.
7. Van Keer, R. L., Deschepper, R., Francke, A. L., Huyghens, L. & Bilsen, J. (2015) Conflicts between healthcare professionals and families of a multi-ethnic patient population during critical care: an ethnographic study. *Crit Care*, 19, 441.
8. Wilkinson, D. (2017) Conscientious Non-objection in Intensive Care. *Camb Q Healthc Ethics*, 26, 132–142.
9. Meller, S. & Barclay, S. (2011) Mediation: an approach to intractable disputes between parents and paediatricians. *Arch Dis Child*, 96, 619–621.
10. Mulcahy, L. (2000) Mediating medical negligence claims. *Amicus Curiae*, 30:21–22.
11. Forbat, L., Simons, J., Sayer, C., Davies, M. & Barclay, S. (2017) Training paediatric healthcare staff in recognising, understanding and managing conflict with patients and families: findings from a survey on immediate and 6-month impact. *Arch Dis Child*, 102, 250–254.
12. Ubel, P. A. & Arnold, R. M. (1995) The unbearable rightness of bedside rationing. Physician duties in a climate of cost containment. *Arch Intern Med*, 155, 1837–1842.
13. Daniels, N. (2008) *Just health: meeting health needs fairly*. Cambridge, Cambridge University Press.
14. Wilkinson, D., and J. Savulescu. (2017) After Charlie Gard: ethically ensuring access to innovative treatment. *Lancet* 390 (10094):540-542. doi: 10.1016/S0140-6736(17)32125-6.
15. Russell, J., Greenhalgh, T., Burnett, A. & Montgomery, J. (2011) "No decisions about us without us"? Individual healthcare rationing in a fiscal ice age. *BMJ*, 342, d3279.
16. Wilkinson, D. & Savulescu, J. (2012) A costly separation between withdrawing and withholding treatment in intensive care. *Bioethics*, 26, 32–48.
17. Sulmasy, D. P. & Sugarman, J. (1994) Are withholding and withdrawing therapy always morally equivalent? *J Med Ethics*, 20, 218–222; discussion 223–224.
18. Andriolo, B. N., Andriolo, R. B., Saconato, H., Atallah, A. N. & Valente, O. (2015) Early versus late tracheostomy for critically ill patients. *Cochrane Database Syst Rev*, 1, CD007271.

19. Wood, D., McShane, P. & Davis, P. (2012) Tracheostomy in children admitted to paediatric intensive care. *Arch Dis Child*, 97, 866–869.

20. Overman, A. E., Liu, M., Kurachek, S. C., Shreve, M. R., Maynard, R. C., Mammel, M. C., et al. (2013) Tracheostomy for infants requiring prolonged mechanical ventilation: 10 years' experience. *Pediatrics*, 131, e1491–1496.

21. Wilkinson, D., Petrou, S., Savulescu, J. (2018) Rationing potentially inappropriate treatment in newborn intensive care in developed countries. *Semin Fetal Neonatal Med* 23 (1):52-58.

22. Wilkinson, D., Petrou, S., Savulescu, J. (2018) Expensive care? Resource-based thresholds for potentially inappropriate treatment in intensive care. *Monash Bioeth Rev* (forthcoming). doi: 10.1007/s40592-017-0075-5.

23. Daniels, N. & Sabin, J. E. (1998) Last chance therapies and managed care. Pluralism, fair procedures, and legitimacy. *Hastings Cent Rep*, 28, 27–41.

24. Romm, C. (2015) Is It Fair to Ask the Internet to Pay Your Hospital Bill? *The Atlantic*. Accessed from <https://www.theatlantic.com/health/archive/2015/03/is-it-fair-to-ask-the-internet-to-pay-your-hospital-bill/387577/>.

25. https://www.thelifeyoucansave.org/impact-calculator

26. Pope, T. (2016) "Texas Advance Directives Act: Nearly a Model Dispute Resolution Mechanism for Intractable Medical Futility Conflicts". *Faculty Scholarship. Paper 378.* accessed from <http://open.mitchellhamline.edu/facsch/378>.

27. Aaronson, B. (2013) A Texas Senate Bill Would Revise the State's End-of-Life Procedure. *New York Times*. accessed from <http://www.nytimes.com/2013/03/31/health/state-senate-bill-would-revise-end-of-life-procedure.html>.

CHAPTER 9

Learning from Charlie Gard

What Should Be Done Next Time?

'Always to have lessons to learn! Oh, I shouldn't like that!'
Alice's Adventures in Wonderland, Lewis Carroll

"'Tis a pitiful tale," said the Bellman, whose face
Had grown longer at every word:
"But, now that you've stated the whole of your case,
More debate would be simply absurd."'
The Hunting of the Snark, Lewis Carroll

In Chapter 3, we described a severe congenital genetic disorder, different from the one that afflicted Charlie Gard, which also causes severe weakness in babies and can lead to them being dependent on life support in intensive care.

Spinal muscular atrophy (SMA) is due to a genetic deletion or mutation of a gene (*SMN1*) that makes an important protein found in the nerves that control muscles. Without this protein (called survival motor neuron), the nerves degenerate, and babies develop progressive muscle weakness. In the severe form, infants develop weakness from birth, or within the first weeks or months of life, though SMA does not affect the brain. The severe form is subdivided into type 'zero' (also called 1A) (newborn or prenatal onset) and type 1 (onset in early infancy). If provided with palliative (comfort-focused) care, the median survival of infants with type 1 SMA is just 7 or 8 months,[1] and few survive for more than 2 years.[2] Alternatively, if breathing support is provided noninvasively (i.e., by mask) or invasively (by tracheostomy), most infants have become dependent on breathing support for more than 16 hours a day by the same age.[3]

We discussed previously some of the court cases in the UK around treatment for infants with SMA (Chapter 3). In those cases, courts sometimes decided that providing ongoing mechanical ventilation for infants with severe SMA was not in their best interests. When there was disagreement between parents and healthcare teams in those cases, treatment was withdrawn, against the wishes of parents.

From the discussions in previous chapters, we have already suggested that the question of best interests in the setting of severe muscular weakness is less clear than some courts and professionals have suggested. This is exactly the sort of case in which there may be reasonable disagreement about what would be best for a child.

However, there is an additional complication that might arise in a future case of treatment disagreement relating to SMA. There are two new experimental treatments for SMA whose benefits are still unclear, but which might offer significant benefit. Important new evidence about both of these treatments was published in the second half of 2017.

Nusinersen is a novel drug that is designed to increase the amounts of survival motor neuron protein. It works via a backup gene for *SMN1*. The backup gene (called *SMN2*) can also make survival motor neuron protein, though it normally doesn't do this very effectively. Children who have more copies of the backup gene have less severe forms of SMA. Nusinersen works on this backup gene to increase the amount of protein made. It is given by repeated injections into the spinal fluid. Several pilot studies of nusinersen had suggested that this treatment could lead to improvement in muscle strength in infants with type 1 SMA, and potentially improve survival. The first randomised trial of nusinersen, published in the *New England Journal of Medicine* in November 2017, studied the treatment in 122 infants, half of whom received the new drug.[4] Infants treated with nusinersen were more likely to develop and achieve motor milestones during the course of the study. Twenty percent of treated infants developed full head control, 10% were able to roll over, 8% were able to sit independently and 1% were able to stand. None of the infants in the control group achieved any of these milestones. The risk of infants either dying or needing to receive permanent breathing support was halved in the treated infants.

The second new proposed treatment for SMA is a gene therapy called scAAV9. This involves a single injection of a modified virus. This is called 'somatic gene therapy' because it affects the developing cells of the body (soma). The virus inserts a copy of the normal *SMN1* gene into the child's DNA. In mice with a form of SMA, the gene therapy had been shown to allow nerve cells and other tissues to produce the survival motor neuron protein. At a higher dose, the gene therapy increased mouse survival from only 15 days to more than 250 days. The first human study of scAAV9 gave the treatment to 15 infants with type 1 SMA and was also published in November 2017.[3] Three infants received a lower dose and did not achieve motor milestones. Twelve infants received a higher dose; nine of these infants were able to sit by the end of the study, and two were able to walk. By the end of the study, none of the 15 treated infants had died, or required permanent mechanical ventilation at an age of 20 months. The study authors compared that to previous reports of infants with similar features – only 8% of such untreated infants were alive at 20 months of age without needing permanent mechanical ventilation.

While the published studies of both of these new drugs look extremely promising, neither is a cure for SMA. There are also considerable uncertainties and downsides. For both drugs, scientific studies at the time of writing have reported follow-up only for the first year or two of life. It is not clear whether the apparent improvement will be sustained, or whether treatment will unmask problems in other tissues and organs.[5] While there were improvements in muscle strength and in need for support, infants still had significant problems. In the scAAV9 study, 5 out of 12 infants still required noninvasive ventilator support at the end of the study; half of the infants needed a gastrostomy or nasogastric feeding tube. In the nusinersen study, 39% of infants who received treatment still died or deteriorated to the point of needing full-time breathing support. There are some very significant practical limitations to nusinersen – it needs to be given via regular, potentially lifelong, injections into the spinal fluid. It is also extremely expensive. One estimate puts the cost at $750,000 per year[6]; another puts the drug cost at £235,000 per year, though the cost would be higher in the first year of treatment, and this does not include the hospital costs incurred in administering the specialised treatment.[7] At this point, the cost of scAAV9 is not clear. It has not yet been approved for clinical use by regulatory authorities. Whether there could be long-term serious side effects of the gene therapy is unknown.

At the time of writing, nusinersen is available in the UK for children who meet specific eligibility criteria through a compassionate use 'Expanded Access Programme', whereby the drug is provided free by the manufacturer for the life of a child, while the NHS has agreed to cover the hospital costs of administering the treatment.[8] However, as the following hypothetical example illustrates, this scheme does not cover all situations. For example, it excludes some of the most severely affected infants.

Hypothetical case of infant 'S'

S is born in late 2017. He is a long-awaited first child to his parents, Stefan and Janeczka, who are academics who migrated to the UK from Poland several years ago. Routine ultrasounds during pregnancy were normal; however, there are problems apparent immediately after S is born. S makes only a weak cry, is floppy and appears to have poor breathing effort. He is admitted to the neonatal intensive care unit, where doctors initially suspect that he may have birth asphyxia. He is put on a ventilator within the first hours of birth because of respiratory failure. However, further tests raise the possibility that S has an underlying disorder of his muscles or nerves. Brain scans and brain electrical tracings are normal. He has further assessment by specialist neurology and genetics teams. Molecular genetic testing reveals that S has a deletion of the *SMN1* gene, confirming a diagnosis of severe (neonatal onset) type 1A SMA. He has a single copy of the backup gene *SMN2*.[a]

S's doctors explain the diagnosis to his devastated parents. The medical teams explain that S has the most severe neonatal form of SMA. There is no available cure, and all affected infants with this condition die in infancy. The doctors mention that, while an experimental treatment is sometimes helpful in other forms of the condition, it is not an option for S. (The Expanded Access Programme for nusinersen excludes infants with type 1A SMA and only a single copy of *SMN2*.) The doctors feel that continuing breathing support is merely prolonging a poor quality of life for S and is not in S's best interests. They seek the parents' permission to withdraw life support and allow S to die.

Stefan and Janeczka find this news difficult to accept. They do some reading on the internet and find descriptions of long-term survival in some children with type 1A SMA. They have also read the recent papers describing the effect of scAAV9 and nusinersen. They refuse to allow the doctors to withdraw treatment. They argue that S should be allowed a trial of at least one of these drugs (preferably both). If the doctors in England will not allow this, they wish to take him overseas to receive the treatment.

Applying the model

How would our model for treatment disagreement apply in this hypothetical case?

In this case, there has been a policy assessment that relates to one of the experimental treatments that Stefan and Janeczka are seeking for their son. The NHS commissioning policy for nusinersen, published in August 2017, allows the drug to be given as part of the Expanded Access Programme (supplied by the drug company) for infants with type 1 SMA. However, that policy specifically excludes infants with the more severe type 1A genetic subtype affecting S.

> '*SMA1A (also called SMA0) is a special category by virtue of its extreme severity, and which requires discussion with the parents on the basis that SMA1A infants are very unlikely to respond to Nusinersen. Thus nusinersen EAP will not be an appropriate intervention for SMA 1A infants.*'[10]

The next option would be whether there is a relevant clinical trial that S could enrol in. If so, that might allow access to one or both of the experimental therapies. However, this may well not be possible. Most of the clinical trials to date have restricted eligibility to infants with two copies of the *SMN2* gene. (In Chapter 5, we argued that it is ethically flawed to exclude

---

[a]Infants with the neonatal onset (type zero/1A) form usually have only one copy of SMN2.[9]

patients from trials with the most severe forms of disease and who will certainly die without treatment.)

If the policy excludes treatment for S, and there are no trials, that might seem to be the end of the question. However, while the national policy about nusinersen assessment is highly relevant, the question is whether existing evidence can be applied to a specific infant whose condition and outlook may be different from those who were studied in trials. Moreover, there is a further question (not addressed by the policy) whether this treatment could be available if privately funded. This is exactly the type of situation where the process model that we described for reviewing treatment would be valuable.

In this case, then, the clinical team asks for S's case to be reviewed urgently by the Critical Care Triage and Treatment Review Panel (CTRP). As described in the previous chapter, this is an independent body (i.e., distinct from a hospital ethics committee) that would have representation from expert health professionals, as well as incorporating ethicists and lay representatives. Its aim would be to provide an impartial, fair, non–court-based process for arbitrating disagreement about specialised medical treatment. After receiving the referral, the panel asks the clinical team to explore the feasibility of providing the desired treatment as a time-limited trial. If there is a way to commence treatment while the review process is being undertaken, that might conceivably provide useful information about how well it is tolerated, as well as any early signs of effectiveness. There is some urgency to commence treatment, given that SMA is a degenerative disorder, and some of the available evidence suggests that earlier treatment is more likely to be effective.[11] In this case, nusinersen is already available, and it is possible that the drug company could be persuaded to provide it on a compassionate basis for a short trial period in S (pending further review). By contrast, scAAV9 is unlikely to be available outside a trial as it is not yet approved for clinical use. S has a first injection of nusinersen the day prior to the CTRP meeting.

As in the case of Charlie Gard, there are two linked questions: should intensive care for S be continued, and should he be provided with experimental treatment? The CTRP decides to address those questions separately. It seeks evidence from the clinical team currently caring for S, both about his clinical condition and, importantly, why they feel that further treatment is not in S's best interests. The panel also asks to hear directly from any health professionals who would support providing treatment for S, and about their reasons for reaching a different conclusion. Finally, they hear from Stefan and Janeczka about their views on further intensive care and experimental treatment for S.

In S's case, there is disagreement about what would be best for him. As discussed in Chapter 7, the important question is whether this disagreement is reasonable or unreasonable. We previously suggested some practical tests for reasonable disagreement – whether the professionals advocating treatment had relevant experience and specific knowledge of the patient's condition, as well as whether they would personally be prepared to take over care and provide treatment. We also indicated more substantive criteria for reasonable disagreement: are those supporting treatment able to provide clear reasons in favour of their view? Do the views appear to be sensitive to changes in evidence? Are they based on reasons that are acceptable within the legal and ethical framework for decisions about children in the UK?

The CTRP hears from the medical team currently caring for S. They describe their grave concern for his quality of life, and worry that he is suffering, despite being unable to show outward signs of distress. They point out that the requested experimental treatments have never been tried in S's genetic variant of SMA. They further note that nusinersen relies on using the backup gene *SMN2*, and S has only a single copy of this gene. S's condition is both more severe than any of the children previously treated with the drug and less likely to respond to the drug. They feel that continuing intensive care to try this treatment would likely do more harm than good.

On the other side, the CTRP hears from a US paediatric rehabilitation specialist with considerable experience in the care of children with SMA, including children with the severe type 1A form that afflicts S. The specialist explains that children with this condition are often able to be managed with noninvasive face-mask breathing support at home and can survive into adulthood. Those children and their families, he argues, report having happy and fulfilling lives, despite their challenges.

The specialist is not able to attend the panel meeting because of pressing clinical commitments. However, a UK paediatrician who has trained with the US specialist has reviewed S in person and gives evidence. She acknowledges that S's condition is at the most severe end of the spectrum of SMA. However, she is hopeful, given the recent experience with experimental drugs, that S's muscle strength would improve enough for him to come off the ventilator and be managed with noninvasive support.

Stefan and Janeczka, meanwhile, make the case that they want to give S the chance of this treatment. They do not wish to keep him alive on life support at all costs. They hope that he might be able to transition to noninvasive breathing support, as described by the US expert. If he shows no sign of improvement, they would not wish S to have long-term mechanical ventilation and would seek to withdraw life support.

What would the CTRP decide in this case? Given the relatively low chance of benefit from experimental treatment, and the scarcity and cost of paediatric intensive care beds, we think that it is inevitable that the CTRP would decide that continued intensive care cannot be provided for S within the public healthcare system. It is also not possible to publicly fund experimental treatment for S as there is no available evidence about the cost-effectiveness of this treatment.

However, the panel is divided when it comes to the question of S's best interests. Some panel members are persuaded by the current clinical team that S may be suffering, and that his chance of improvement with treatment is very small. They do not support the parents' request. However, other members of the panel feel that there is a reasonable case for providing a time-limited trial of treatment for S. They are convinced that the specialist who reviewed S was sincerely motivated by S's wellbeing, and that, while untested, the treatment could be of benefit. Accordingly, the CTRP decides that there is reasonable dissensus about treatment. If S's family are able to fund treatment, it would be ethical to provide continued intensive care and a trial of nusinersen. The panel recommends that any intensive care unit proposing to treat S consider the availability of intensive care beds and provide treatment as a time-limited trial with prespecified endpoints. If private funding for S's treatment is not available, life support should be withdrawn.

After the panel meeting, Stefan and Janeczka's family in Poland offer financial support to the family to enable them to take him to the US. While S's current doctors disagree, they respect the CTRP's decision and decide not to appeal against it. While awaiting transfer, the UK hospital continues to provide treatment in intensive care, as well as further injections of nusinersen supplied by the drug company. S is flown to the US for further treatment 2 weeks later. His family are still waiting to hear whether they will be able to obtain compassionate access to scAAV9.

This hypothetical case of disagreement is based on a real medical condition and real experimental treatments. While we are unaware of any current cases with the features that we have described, we suggest that it is highly plausible that disagreement in a case like this will arise in a UK or other hospital in the near future. The case is designed to summarise and illustrate the lessons that we have learned from the Charlie Gard case. It does not prove in itself that our approach is the right one. The same outcome might be possible another way.

As noted in the last chapter, it would be important for clinicians to spend time with Stefan and Janeczka and to see if agreement can be reached. It would be important to have an open mind and to look at the information that they have found, to see whether it applies to S. It may be helpful for clinicians to seek an external second opinion or mediation if disagreement persists. It is possible, then, that in a real version of the case of infant S, his doctors would agree to Stefan and Janeczka's request for nusinersen, or would allow S to travel to the US. There might be no need for dispute resolution. Alternatively, a rapid court hearing might be possible and might have decided in S's parents favour, with the result that further treatment is deemed to be in S's best interests.

Nevertheless, where agreement cannot be reached, we suggest that the process we have described for resolving disagreements has several obvious advantages over the existing process in countries like the UK. It draws on important lessons learned from the Charlie Gard case.

It may allow decisions to be reached in a way that is more timely, less adversarial and less public. It explicitly allows consideration of limited resources to be taken into account in decisions. It draws on relevant medical and ethical expertise. Importantly, given the overall theme of this book, it incorporates the concept of reasonable disagreement into a framework that allows parents to choose medical treatment for their child on the basis of their understanding of what would be best – while also preventing parents from making harmful choices. Finally, we suggest that this process is unlikely to result in the prolonged, bitter and painful dispute seen in the Gard case, where ultimately no one was the winner.

Health professionals sometimes feel dispirited or depressed when they encounter patients or families who do not share the health professional's viewpoint about treatment. Some doctors appear affronted that the patient/family might not accept their view or advice – it is a rejection or dismissal of their expertise. Others perceive disagreement as a sign of failure – that they have failed to communicate clearly or adequately, and that if only they had approached discussions differently, disagreement would not have arisen. Yet, for reasons that should be clear from the preceding chapters, disagreement does not need to be seen as a negative. Indeed, it can be a way to make progress. Decisions about medical treatment depend on more than just knowledge of the medical facts. Value-based disagreements are part of living in diverse progressive communities. So, in a sense, disagreement is a good thing – it is a sign of a pluralistic and tolerant society. However, it is also a sign of a pluralistic society (rather than a relativistic one) that we recognise limits to reasonable disagreement. The important ethical issue – the one that professionals and society should be focusing on as a measure of success or failure – is how well we respond to that disagreement. Can we deal with dissensus? Can we agree to disagree?

The Charlie Gard case, the springboard for discussion throughout this book, represents a paradigm case of contemporary medical/family disagreement about treatment. It provides an important opportunity to consider the strengths and limitations of existing ways of responding to disagreement. The kind of dispute present in the case of Charlie Gard will now only multiply, as science progresses, more experimental treatments become available and society finds itself unable to provide all treatments that could be of benefit or could be desired. Moreover, parents and patients are and will continue to be empowered (and simultaneously disempowered) by the internet and their ready access to information about possible treatments. The internet will also make it much easier for families to appeal to public opinion and to raise funds in an attempt to fund treatment.

Doubtless, some readers of this book will not have been convinced by the arguments that we have set out here or by the model that we have proposed. They may prefer some variation of the status quo, or some other alternative way of dealing with treatment disputes. We would not expect everyone to have identical views on these questions of how to balance the interests of children, parents and wider society. Indeed, we should not expect agreement on this, given the central arguments of the book.

However, we suggest that everyone who has read this book can agree that there is a need for sensitive, rational debate within our community about how to fairly address disagreements about treatment between health professionals and families. That debate cannot, now, help poor Charlie Gard. It can, though, help current and future children with serious illnesses. It can support their families to access desired treatment, within limits. It can help health professionals to be able to advocate for the best interests of their patients and to maintain relationships with families (even if not always seeing eye to eye). It can help society to understand what is at stake, why these disagreements are so difficult, so vexed, and so inevitable.

> *'Then, silence. Some fancied they heard in the air*
> *A weary and wandering sigh.'*
>
> THE HUNTING OF THE SNARK, LEWIS CARROLL

References

1. Gregoretti, C., Ottonello, G., Chiarini Testa, M. B., Mastella, C., Rava, L., Bignamini, E., et al. (2013) Survival of patients with spinal muscular atrophy type 1. *Pediatrics*, 131, e1509-14.
2. Kolb, S. J., Coffey, C. S., Yankey, J. W., Krosschell, K., Arnold, W. D., Rutkove, S. B., et al. (2017) Natural history of infantile-onset spinal muscular atrophy. *Ann Neurol*, 82, 883-891.
3. Mendell, J. R., Al-Zaidy, S., Shell, R., Arnold, W. D., Rodino-Klapac, L. R., Prior, T. W., et al. (2017) Single-dose gene-replacement therapy for spinal muscular atrophy. *N Engl J Med*, 377, 1713-1722.
4. Finkel, R. S., Mercuri, E., Darras, B. T., Connolly, A. M., Kuntz, N. L., Kirschner, J., et al. (2017) Nusinersen versus Sham Control in Infantile-Onset Spinal Muscular Atrophy. *N Engl J Med* 377:1723-1732.
5. Tizzano, E. F. & Finkel, R. S. (2017) Spinal muscular atrophy: A changing phenotype beyond the clinical trials. *Neuromuscul Disord*, 27, 883-889.
6. van der Ploeg, A. T. (2017) The dilemma of two innovative therapies for spinal muscular atrophy. *N Engl J Med*, 377, 1786-1787.
7. http://www.smasupportuk.org.uk/blog/research/biogen-announces-european-ex-factory-list-price-for-nusinersen
8. (2017, 18 October 2017). *'The UK Expanded Access Programme for Nusinersen for Children with SMA Type 1.'* from <http://www.smasupportuk.org.uk/the-uk-expanded-access-programme-for-nusinersen-for-children-with-sma-type-1>.
9. Arnold, W. D., Kassar, D. & Kissel, J. T. (2015) Spinal muscular atrophy: diagnosis and management in a new therapeutic era. *Muscle Nerve*, 51, 157-67.
10. NHS England. (2017, August 4, 2017). *'Urgent Clinical Commissioning Policy Statement: Nusinersen for genetically confirmed Spinal Muscular Atrophy (SMA) type 1 for eligible patients under the Expanded Access Programme (EAP).'* from <https://www.england.nhs.uk/wp-content/uploads/2017/08/clinical-comm-pol-nusinersen-170018P.pdf>.

Wilkinson's view

Why further medical treatment for Charlie Gard would have been unethical

The prospect of losing a child is terrible, beyond words. I have sat with parents in the terrifying, awful stillness after telling them that I thought their child was going to die. In that silence, it feels as though the earth has stopped spinning. For those parents, nothing, from that moment, can ever be the same.

It is completely normal, completely understandable for parents to struggle to believe that news, to think that it must be a mistake, to hope for a miracle and to want to hold on to their son or daughter. Anyone reading of the plight of Charlie's parents would feel enormous sympathy for them. Many might feel that in the same circumstances they would feel the same way, would feel the same need to fight for their child, no matter what, until the very end.

The sad truth, though, is that despite all our technology, all our medical advances, there are some illnesses that medicine cannot cure, cannot make better. There are real limits to the capacity of medicine to help or to heal. At the same time medical machines, drugs and procedures have real (almost unlimited) potential to harm, to hurt and to make sick and dying patients miserable. Sometimes, despite our best intentions, medicine causes suffering and discomfort while merely prolonging the dying of a child or an adult.

It is often difficult to know whether it is the right thing to do to continue life-prolonging treatment in the hope of improvement, or whether to stop trying to prolong life and to focus on the patient's comfort for the time that they have remaining. In many cases, there may be more than one reasonable course of action, and health professionals should be guided by the wishes of a child's parents. They should provide treatment, even if that goes against their personal assessment of what would be best for the child. Indeed, much of this book has been dedicated to the complexity of decisions and to understanding why there can often be a range of different reasonable points of view. Yet, in some cases, it is abundantly clear that treatment offers no realistic chance of helping a child, while also having a real prospect of harming them. In that situation, health professionals have a fundamental ethical obligation to safeguard the interests of the child. They *should* refuse to provide or continue treatment. It would be unethical to do otherwise. That was the reason why the doctors at Great Ormond Street Hospital opposed continued intensive care for Charlie Gard and took the case to the court. It was the reason why the courts (four different courts) supported the decision not to allow his transfer overseas for nucleoside treatment. It is the reason why I was convinced that this was the right decision.

Treatment was not in Charlie's best interests

Julian Savulescu argues (in Appendix 2, below) that it was potentially in Charlie's interests to have continued treatment in intensive care, and to have received a trial of nucleoside therapy. In particular, he contends that there was sufficient uncertainty about the central medical and ethical questions that (so long as they were able to pay for it) Charlie's parents' wishes should have been respected.

149

There are three key areas of disagreement between us. Julian argues that quality of life is too difficult and contentious to justify limiting treatment in Charlie's case, that Charlie was not suffering (or his suffering was likely insignificant) and that, in the face of a very small chance of benefit, it would have been in Charlie's best interests to receive the requested treatment.

I will argue that a quality of life judgment was possible in Charlie's case, that there was a real possibility of Charlie suffering from continued intensive care and that it was considerably more likely that Charlie would be harmed by intensive care than that he would be helped. Complete certainty is impossible. However, based on the information and evidence available at the time, it would not have been right to agree to his parents' requests for further intensive care.

Why did the doctors feel so strongly that treatment was not in Charlie's best interests? There are several elements to that.

QUALITY OF LIFE

Charlie was severely ill, on life support in intensive care. His mitochondrial problem caused severe muscle weakness, and he was completely paralysed. He could not open his eyes and was deaf. There was also evidence that the disorder was affecting his brain: electrical recordings of his brain showed very abnormal, disordered electrical patterns with frequent subclinical seizures, a pattern referred to as 'severe epileptic encephalopathy'. It was impossible to know whether Charlie was aware of anything around him. However, other children with similar electrical patterns of brain activity have minimal or no awareness. In that situation, life support machines were keeping Charlie alive, but were not benefiting him in any meaningful way.

Of course, quality of life assessments are fraught and difficult. There can be a range of different views about quality of life. Julian highlights the philosophical complexity of assessing wellbeing, as well as the controversial nature of a judgment that someone else's life is 'not worth living'. There are very good reasons to be extremely cautious about making such judgments and to pay particular attention to the views of parents and to those of people with disabilities. However, taking great care about such assessments does not mean that they should never be made, or that any view of parents about their child's quality of life should be accepted uncritically. Imagine, for example, that parents of a child with Down syndrome decided that they did not wish their child to have surgery for a treatable abnormality and would prefer that the child die. They might point to the lack of philosophical agreement on theories of wellbeing, or even to the views of some philosophers that a life with moderate intellectual disability is not a life worth living. Yet, it is clear to almost all readers, I suspect, that it would be wrong to go along with these parents' views about quality of life. As has been pointed out several times in this book, pluralism is not the same thing as relativism. While there may not be a single 'right answer' to the question of how we should think about wellbeing, or what would be a life worth living, there can be wrong answers.

In 2013, in my book *Death or Disability? The 'Carmentis machine' and decision-making for critically ill children,* I focussed specifically on the question of quality of life for children with severe brain problems.[1] I looked at when, if ever, a child's brain problem would be so severe that intensive care should not be continued or provided, even if parents wished it to be. In that book, 4 years before the Gard case, I argued that the combination of very severe cognitive, movement and sensory problems along with ongoing painful illness or medical interventions would be the clearest case where treatment would not be in a child's interests.[1] Why think this? Drawing on the metaphor that we described in Chapter 3 of a set of scales, this situation seems to be one where a child's condition removes all, or almost all, of the benefits of life for the child.

This seems clear whichever philosophical theory of wellbeing we adopt. On a hedonic theory (life goes well if we experience more pleasure than pain), it did not appear that Charlie was able to experience any pleasure at all. He could perhaps be aware of his parents' presence through touch or smell, but he could not hear their voices or see them. If we adopt a desire-based theory, it seems that Charlie was unable to develop any desires or preferences because of his severe brain dysfunction. There are different lists of objective goods; however, many of the things that are present across different lists are closely related to learning, awareness and cognitive function. For example, such lists often include communication, knowledge, aesthetic appreciation, the development of deep reciprocal relationships, the achievement of goals or ambitions. Yet, none of these appeared to be available to Charlie.

Here, the combination of different forms of severe disability is highly relevant. Someone with blindness and deafness, but who has normal learning and movement, can learn to appreciate the world through their other senses. There can still be enormous benefits and value of their life (for them) – as famously evident in the life of Helen Keller. Alternatively, a child with a severe learning disability may still be able to develop deep and valuable relationships with those around them, may be able to communicate nonverbally and may experience a range of sensory pleasures, as well as pleasure in learning and gaining new skills. There is also important evidence from those with severe physical impairment – even profound forms such as quadriplegia or locked-in syndrome. Such individuals often report high levels of personal wellbeing, despite their physical limitations.[2] These are all examples of humans' capacity to adapt to illness or impairment and to find value in life despite adversity. However, the combination of severe or profound impairments of different types makes it very difficult, and perhaps impossible, to compensate or adapt. That is why I have argued that, in this situation, doctors would potentially be justified in declining to keep a child alive.

Charlie's condition, by the time that nucleoside therapy was being contemplated, had left him in a state of profound weakness, with very abnormal brain function and sensory impairment. His condition, then, was much more severe than some of the cases discussed earlier in this book. Jonathan Simms, the adolescent with Creutzfeldt-Jakob disease discussed in Chapter 5, was able to recognise and respond to his family, listen to music and enjoy watching games of soccer on the television.[3] Infant MB, who had profound muscle weakness from spinal muscular atrophy (Chapter 3), was thought to be able to appreciate and gain pleasure from stories that were read to him, or from watching DVDs.[4]

Importantly, Charlie's parents in the court hearing accepted that Charlie's current quality of life was not good – they did not wish to prolong his life as it was.

SUFFERING

I have argued that, in Charlie's case, there was little benefit to him in keeping him alive. But what of the other side of the scales? If there is no reason to think that a child is in pain or discomfort, it is hard to see what would be wrong in prolonging their life with medical treatment (setting aside any issue of limited resources).

The medical professionals who cared for Charlie were concerned that he was suffering and would be harmed by continuing life support. (As far as was known, the nucleoside treatment had few side effects.) In large part, that seemed to be because they were aware of the unpleasantness of keeping children or adults alive in intensive care. Despite the best efforts of doctors and nurses to minimise invasive procedures and tests, and to use drugs and other measures to manage symptoms, being on life support in intensive care is often painful and uncomfortable. However, as noted by Julian and other commentators, there are plenty of children who receive treatment (sometimes very prolonged treatment) in intensive care. Extremely premature infants, sometimes with relatively low chances of survival, may be ventilated and have multiple invasive procedures over a period of 3 months or more. Ethicists and doctors do not normally seem to be worried about the suffering inflicted on children by being in intensive care.

But the situation of most children in intensive care is different from the situation that faced Charlie. Even if unpleasant, the pain and discomfort of life support is worth enduring if a child is going to get better and ultimately be able to be discharged home. For example, in a recent cohort, 36% of extremely premature infants born at 22–24 weeks' gestation survived to at least age 18 months (and more than 50% of survivors had no neurosensory disability).[5] But where there isn't any real chance that the child will improve, the patient has to endure the side effects of intensive care without any benefits.

In Charlie's case, there was some disagreement about whether he was suffering. His parents spent hours at his bedside and felt that they knew him well. They did not believe that he was in pain. Yet, one of the sad features of Charlie's illness was that it rendered him completely paralysed and unable to show any outward sign of anything. He could not indicate his needs, he could not even cry if he were uncomfortable. The nurses and doctors looking after Charlie would have been aware that other children in the intensive care unit on life support show signs of pain and discomfort, at least some of the time. They would have suspected that Charlie would have similar periods – though because of his paralysis, they could not tell when.

Charlie's situation, then, was different from that of the brain-dead children discussed in Chapter 2 (infant A and Jahi McMath). In those cases, there is very good reason to think that they had or have zero capacity for suffering. While there may be no benefit to them of continuing somatic support, there is equally no harm.

For Charlie, there were two possibilities.

One possibility was that Charlie's brain was so severely affected that he did not even experience pain. Perhaps he was genuinely in something akin to a persistent vegetative state or a state of brain death. (He did not apparently fulfil criteria for brain death.) If that were the case, it might not be harmful to Charlie to continue intensive care and to receive nucleoside therapy. At the same time, if his brain were that severely affected by mitochondrial DNA depletion syndrome (MDDS) that he experienced no pain at all, it would be even more improbable that nucleoside treatment would help.

However, another very real possibility was that Charlie was at least intermittently aware of his surroundings, perhaps in something like a 'minimally conscious state'. If that were the case, there was a real worry that some of the time he would be distressed, agitated or unhappy, but paralysed. Neuroimaging studies suggest that severely brain-injured adults in a minimally conscious state are able to perceive pain.[6] With no easy way to detect pain in Charlie, it would be hard to console him or treat his pain.

UNCERTAINTY

The court found that nucleoside treatment for Charlie would be futile. However, as Julian persuasively argues below, this appears to be a mistake. There is a key difference between there being no evidence that something will work and there being clear evidence that it will not work. Brain scans did not show, indeed could not show, 'irreversible' damage to his brain. The question of whether brain damage is reversible is a prediction about future brain function and whether it will improve. It can't simply be read from a scan. It depends on experience from past patients who have received similar treatment. But of course, there weren't any of those.

It was not possible to be certain that nucleoside therapy would not lead to any improvement in Charlie. It would not have been 'futile'. On the strictest definitions of futility, there are very few situations in medicine where it is possible to be certain that treatment absolutely cannot work.

However, everyone involved in assessing Charlie (including Professor Hirano) agreed that it was very unlikely that nucleoside therapy would lead to any significant improvement. Why did they believe this?

All previous children with Charlie's severe condition had died. Charlie had progressively and inexorably deteriorated over time due to MDDS. By January 2017, there was evidence of severe epileptic encephalopathy. Nucleoside treatment for Charlie's condition had never been tried in animal models, never been tried in other children and, importantly, had (in other forms of MDDS) never been shown to improve brain problems. Even in children with the milder muscle-only form of MDDS, nucleoside treatment wasn't a cure, it wasn't a magic bullet. It led to some improvement in muscle strength, but most children remained dependent on breathing support. It seemed extremely unlikely in Charlie's much more severe situation, with established severe brain problems, that the treatment would make any difference at all.

But so what? Even if the treatment was unlikely to help Charlie, the alternative, as bluntly noted by Professor Hirano, was death. Julian points out, that faced with certain death, many adults might be willing to take the gamble of several months of intensive care and an experimental treatment, even if the odds of benefit were tiny. He contends that this would be a reasonable choice by an adult and potentially in their interests. Accordingly, we should think it a reasonable option for Charlie Gard, and potentially in his interests.

In Chapter 3, we discussed some of the challenges of assessing best interests in the face of uncertainty. People have different attitudes to risks, and place different weights on the best- or worst-case scenario. Whether or not it is worth undergoing an intervention that has only a small chance of benefit depends a lot on how unpleasant or risky it would be (which would take us back to the suffering question, discussed previously). It may also depend on someone's perspective. From a parent's point of view, they are focussed on the child in front of them and face the devastating prospect of losing their child. The statistics are, in a sense, meaningless to them. Their child will die or will recover. It is completely understandable that they would seize any chance of avoiding that terrible loss.

Yet from the professionals' point of view, and from the point of view of society, it is important to step back from an individual child to think about what the implications would be of allowing parents to subject their children to very unpleasant treatments that have only a very small chance of helping them. If doctors or judges allow those decisions, that will mean that many children will suffer the side effects and harms of treatment for only a very few children to see any benefit. As noted in Chapter 3, if the chance of Charlie benefiting from nucleoside therapy were 1 in 10,000, that would mean that similar treatment choices would harm 9999 children for every child that they help.

This argument has some overlap with other so-called 'collective action' problems (for example, climate change, voting or littering). While the impact of any individual act is small, the total effect will be substantial if everybody takes that action. For example, you may be wondering whether to go to the trouble of visiting the polling booth on election day. Perhaps you feel that it is important which party is elected, but that it does not matter if you decide not to vote – the chance of your individual vote making the difference between one party winning or losing in an election is remote. However, if everyone reasoned the same way, that would make a very large difference.

A particularly apt example, described by philosopher Derek Parfit, is a thought experiment he called the 'Harmless Torturers'. Parfit imagined that a torture machine that administered a large and painful electrical charge was replaced by many machines operated by 1000 different torturers who each administered an imperceptible charge (1/1000th of the previous amount).[7] None of the individual torturers was harming anyone perceptibly, but together they predictably caused terrible pain. We shouldn't allow them to administer their tiny shocks because we know what will happen if they do. Low probability treatments in intensive care might seem very similar to 'harmless torture'.

Of course, the decision faced by parents of a dying child is not the same. They do not intend to harm their child. Nor do their choices combine or interact with others in the way that votes combine, or that mini-shocks add up. But it is similar in the sense that a decision that might be understandable and rational from the point of view of any individual becomes unwise and obviously harmful when seen as a general rule or principle.

This is not a mere theoretical point about statistics and abstract philosophical theories. In the intensive care unit where I work, every week there are some infants whose outcome is uncertain, but who my colleagues and I judge are unlikely to survive. Reflecting back on similar infants over the past year, many of the infants in that category did die, often after many weeks or even months of invasive and unpleasant treatment. However, some of the infants also survived.[a] In the face of uncertainty, those parents asked us to continue intensive care, and, because of the degree of uncertainty, we provided that treatment. But sometimes the chance of benefit seems even smaller, and the risks overwhelming. Several years ago, I cared for an infant who had been in intensive care on a ventilator for 6 months. She had deteriorated despite maximal treatment, and sadly we had exhausted all ideas about further treatments to help. Specialists from a number of different departments reviewed her, and none of them, nor any of my colleagues, believed that she would survive. Her parents, though, would not agree to withdraw treatment. The infant lingered for weeks more in the intensive care unit. Despite our best efforts to provide pain relief, she had become tolerant to many of our medications – she often appeared uncomfortable or in pain. Eventually, as predicted, she deteriorated further, and died after more than 8 months in the intensive care unit.

If it were justified for doctors to refuse to provide treatments that have a real prospect of harming children and only a low chance of benefit, that obviously raises difficult questions about how small a chance of benefit would count. There is no straightforward answer to that question. Should it be 10%, or 1% or lower? It will depend on how harmful the treatment is (again circling back to the earlier question of suffering). In my book *Death or Disability*, I adopted the legal standard of clear and convincing evidence.[1] In the courtroom, as in the neonatal intensive care unit (NICU), it is rarely possible to be 100% certain – but decisions still have to be made. If there is clear and convincing evidence that treatment would harm an infant or child, it should not be provided, even if parents request it. My view in the Gard case was that there appeared to be such evidence, and that it was both clear and, to those who reviewed it in detail, convincing.

REASONABLE DISAGREEMENT

The recurring theme throughout this book has been that of reasonable disagreement, and the importance of acknowledging and respecting differing viewpoints about difficult and contested questions of value. Where there is reasonable disagreement (and where there are no questions of limited resources), we have argued that parents' wishes should be respected.

In the case of Charlie Gard, there were such differing points of view. There were some professionals in Italy and in the US who supported the option of nucleoside treatment and were prepared to provide the treatment if Charlie were transferred to their centres. There were also some ethicists who defended that option and felt that the court decision was flawed. Julian, below, articulates a strong case in favour of allowing Charlie to undergo such treatment.

---

[a]US Neonatologist Bill Meadow powerfully quantified this sort of anecdotal evidence in a series of studies from the NICU.[8,9] Approximately 50% of extremely premature infants, where more than one professional believed on more than 1 day that the infant would die before discharge, ultimately died without going home.

However, some of the conditions of reasonableness that we have set out in this book did not seem to be met at the time that Charlie's case was being actively debated in the courts. It wasn't clear whether Professor Hirano had all of the necessary information about Charlie's current condition to reach an informed decision about what would be best for him. In the High Court hearing, he admitted that it was difficult for him to assess Charlie from a distance:

> 'Perhaps, if I were there, I would support [the Great Ormond Street Hospital's plan to withdraw treatment]. Not seeing the child, not seeing progression, it's difficult for me to make an assessment.' para 99[10]

While Professor Hirano was able to provide the nucleoside treatment, he noted that he would defer a decision about provision of life support to 'ICU people'. There were no submissions, however, from intensive care specialists in the US. All of the intensive care experts from the UK (and all the other medical specialists who had reviewed him in person) had concluded that continuing treatment and nucleoside therapy was not in his interests.

It was also unclear whether Professor Hirano or, at a later stage, the other specialists (for example from the Vatican hospital in Rome) who provided support for the requested treatment were motivated by values that are not relevant within the context of UK legal decision-making. For example, in Chapter 7 we argued that 'reasonable dissensus' would not be present if professionals defended treatment on the basis of a belief that parents should always be the ultimate decision makers about treatment or on the basis of a strong sanctity of life view.

This is not to cast aspersions on the views of these experts. It is possible that they knew all of the relevant facts and were genuinely motivated by concern for Charlie's interests. However, given that they were offering views that were in opposition to those of all of the medical team caring for Charlie, as well as all of the external experts who had examined him, it would have been vital to present evidence to substantiate the reasonableness of their views. It would have been important to be clear about the values underlying their opinions. That evidence was never, to my knowledge, presented.

Conclusions

I have argued that the decision to withdraw life support from Charlie Gard, and not to allow him to be transferred overseas for experimental treatment, was the right decision. It is worth, though, noting some important limitations to this conclusion. I am not a specialist in mitochondrial disease, or in paediatric intensive care. I did not ever review Charlie in person, and I based this assessment only on evidence available in the public domain about his condition. There are highly likely to be relevant features of Charlie's condition and of his case that I do not know, that might make a difference to an assessment of the ethical issues. I cannot, in truth, claim to know what was in Charlie's best interests. I can only present arguments on the basis of the evidence that is and was available.

I should also acknowledge the possibility that I am wrong. Perhaps I have overestimated the chance and nature of suffering that Charlie would have endured from continued intensive care. Perhaps I have underestimated the chance or magnitude of improvement from nucleoside therapy. My own experience as a consultant in newborn intensive care gives me a different perspective on the harms and benefits of treatment – but not necessarily a better perspective than that of a parent of a seriously ill child.

The courts and the media often frame these cases in terms that are black or white. They like clear, unambiguous statements and assessments. They like people to line up on one side or the other. Reality, though is much more messy, more complicated, more grey. Reflecting back on the case of Charlie Gard, more than a year after it first hit the headlines, having debated it at length in print and in person, and having spoken with a wide range of people, medics and non-medics, I feel less sure that I know who was right and who was wrong. In retrospect, I wish that Charlie had received a trial of nucleoside therapy back in January 2017. Even if it had not helped at all, that could not have been worse than the long struggle that followed. It would have saved months of heartache for everyone involved.

These decisions, about life and death, quality versus quantity of life, risks and uncertainty, are awful. All any of us can do, as health professionals, or as judges or as parents, is to try to make the best decision that we can for the child in front of us. In this case, Charlie's doctors and his parents fought so hard because they were each desperately concerned for the wellbeing of an extremely sick child who could not speak for himself. Charlie's parents were doing what they felt was best for him. But so too were the medical team. It would have been much easier for them to simply agree to the requests of Connie Yates and Chris Gard. It would have saved months of heartache for everyone involved. However, the medical team felt strongly that that would be wrong. They believed that they could not ethically provide the treatment that his parents were requesting.

There are problems with relying on courts to resolving these very difficult cases of disagreement, and in this book we have described and defended an alternative approach. We speculated in Chapter 8 on what might have happened in Charlie's case if this approach had been available. Review of Charlie's case by an independent panel might (or might not) have concluded that a time-limited trial of nucleoside therapy was warranted. Nevertheless, at the time of the Gard case, the courts were the only option if doctors and parents could not reach agreement about what would be best for a child. The court, in April 2017 and in the later appeals and hearing in July, could only make decisions on the basis of the evidence and arguments in front of it. With an extremely low chance of improvement, with an apparent prospect of harming Charlie by continuing intensive care and with a level of quality of life that all agreed was unacceptable, the court was bound to conclude, as it did 'with the heaviest of hearts but with complete conviction', that it was in Charlie's best interests to withdraw treatment and to allow him to die.

References

1. Wilkinson, D. (2013) *Death or disability? The Carmentis Machine and treatment decisions for critically ill children.* Oxford, OUP.
2. Bruno, M. A., Bernheim, J. L., Ledoux, D., Pellas, F., Demertzi, A. & Laureys, S. (2011) A survey on self-assessed well-being in a cohort of chronic locked-in syndrome patients: happy majority, miserable minority. *BMJ Open*, 1, e000039.
3. *Simms v An NHS Trust* [2002] EWHC 2734 (Fam) (11 December 2002).
4. *An NHS Trust v MB* [2006] 2 F.L.R. 319.
5. Younge, N., Goldstein, R. F., Bann, C. M., Hintz, S. R., Patel, R. M., Smith, P. B., et al. (2017) Survival and neurodevelopmental outcomes among periviable infants. *N Engl J Med*, 376, 617-628.
6. Boly, M., Faymonville, M. E., Schnakers, C., Peigneux, P., Lambermont, B., Phillips, C., et al. (2008) Perception of pain in the minimally conscious state with PET activation: an observational study. *Lancet Neurol*, 7, 1013-20.
7. Parfit, D. (1984) *Reasons and persons.* Oxford, Oxford University Press. page 80.
8. Meadow, W., Lagatta, J., Andrews, B., Caldarelli, L., Keiser, A., Laporte, J., et al. (2008) Just, in time: ethical implications of serial predictions of death and morbidity for ventilated premature infants. *Pediatrics*, 121, 732–740.
9. Lagatta, J., Andrews, B., Caldarelli, L., Schreiber, M., Plesha-Troyke, S., Meadow, W. (2011) Early neonatal intensive care unit therapy improves predictive power for the outcomes of ventilated extremely low birth weight infants. *J Pediatr*, 159, 384–391.e1.
10. *Great Ormond Street Hospital v Yates & Ors* [2017] EWHC 972 (Fam) (11 April 2017).

Savulescu's view

It was in Charlie Gard's best interests to receive experimental treatment

The basic principle of medical ethics is that treatments which are in the best interests of the patients should be offered or employed (in the case of children and incompetent patients). Best interests means the wellbeing of the patient.

Charlie Gard was born with a severe, incurable, rapidly progressive, lethal genetic disorder. At birth, he was normal, but over a period of weeks he deteriorated. There was no proven or existing treatment for his disorder.

His mother identified nucleoside replacement therapy (NRT) as a potential treatment. Was this in his best interests? The alternative was death. So the essential question was: was the outcome of administering NRT better or worse than death?

If NRT involved a single injection, it clearly should have been tried. But Prof. Hirano, a world expert on mitochondrial replacement therapy, believed a 3-month trial, with associated intensive care, was necessary. If this had been 3 months of agony, then it would depend on what the expected benefit was.

If there was a certainty of full recovery, some people would believe that 3 months of excruciating agony is worth paying for a full, normal life. (Some might disagree.) But in Charlie's case, there was only a low chance of saving his life, and his life would be very disabled at best. It seems unreasonable to impose 3 months of excruciating agony for such a small expected benefit.

However, Charlie was not going to be exposed to 3 months of excruciating agony – he was going to be exposed to 3 months in one of the best intensive care units in the world. Indeed, doctors were even unsure whether he was experiencing any suffering at all, as we shall see.

In my view, the suffering of 3 months of intensive care (which could significantly be reduced by analgesia and sedation) was a price worth paying for a small chance of life of significant disability.[1] NRT, at least early on in Charlie's disease, was worth trying.

Was NRT in Charlie's best interests?

What makes me say that? Here are five arguments.

ARGUMENT 1. CONSISTENCY WITH CURRENT PRACTICE

Many premature infants spend 3 months in the neonatal intensive care unit (NICU) with a very poor prognosis. This is not seen to preclude their treatment. Three months in intensive care is not unusual for a premature infant.

ARGUMENT 2. SUPERIOR TO THE ACTUAL COURSE

Charlie spent 6 months in NICU after the decision not to provide NRT for the sake of procedures, arguments, and legal hearings that had no direct prospect of benefiting him. He suffered all that for nothing.

It might be argued that this long course was unexpected. However, it was clear that all these legal options were open to the parents at the outset. It would have been better to at least have the NRT while these hearings/cases were going on.

ARGUMENT 3. RADICAL UNCERTAINTY

Doctors in the UK were confident that NRT would not help Charlie. That confidence was exaggerated. We really didn't have any rational estimate of what Charlie's chances were of improvement with NRT. At the first hearing, Hirano said that they were 'low but not zero', which seems about as accurate as one could be. When he returned in July with a number of other experts, the chances were put at 10%, but this was based on experience with milder *TK2* deficiency. In reality, these sorts of figures and estimates are relatively meaningless. They are virtually plucking figures out of the air. You wouldn't know until you tried. Markers of response would be crucial to minimising suffering.

ARGUMENT 4. UNIVERSALISABILITY

Universalisability is the moral procedure of putting yourself in the shoes of everyone affected by a decision, also known as the 'Golden Rule': Do unto others as you would have them do unto you.

If it were you, would you want a 3-month trial? I would, and many others would as well. Maybe not everyone, but the fact that some would is some suggestive reason to believe it is beneficial. I look upon it as an 'I have little to lose' option. This is more or less Hirano's view in justifying being prepared to offer it: 'It is unlikely to work, but the alternative is that he will pass away.' (Para 127)[2]

This does not show it is in Charlie Gard's interests because he has never been competent to express such a view. Moreover, it is very difficult to imagine what life would be like in such a situation. But it does indicate that the tradeoff is reasonable, even if some people would reasonably prefer to die.

ARGUMENT 5. CONSISTENCY AND THOUGHT EXPERIMENT.[1]

Consider the following thought experiment which supports the claim that we don't know whether Charlie's life really is 'intolerable'. Imagine that we discovered a baby like Charlie in the US with an identical condition: Charlie Card. However, in Card's case, the condition was picked up soon after birth, and NRT was started as the first symptoms emerged. He has been deeply sedated. He spends nearly all of his day unconscious on a breathing tube. Once every few days, his sedation is lightened to see if there is any improvement in his condition. Doctors have agreed with parents that, if after 6 months of this treatment there is no improvement, they will stop artificial ventilation and allow this baby to die.

Are these doctors acting in a cruel and inhumane manner? Should courts intervene to protect the baby's interests? Is this child abuse? Is this baby being forced to live a life which is not worth living and is intolerable? Should the experimental treatment and artificial ventilation be stopped and this baby be allowed to 'die with dignity' now?

The answer to all these questions is 'no'. Presumably, many babies have been treated in similar circumstances. If it is reasonable to continue treating Charlie Card, it would have been reasonable to start treating Charlie Gard.

These arguments are, admittedly, far from conclusive. There are responses to all of them. However, they do suggest that NRT could reasonably be construed to be in Charlie's best interests. However, the arguments that it was against Charlie's interests – that he would be better off dead than have a 3-month trial of treatment – were even weaker.

Was NRT not in Charlie's best interests?[a]

The courts and the doctors argued that the proposed course of treatment was not in Charlie's interests. There are three ways in which this line of argument might be framed. We have discussed the concept of futility in detail in Chapter 2. It should hopefully already be clear that this concept could not justify withholding NRT.

FUTILITY

The most common argument for further treatment not being in the interests of the patient is that it would be 'futile'. Treatment can be futile for two reasons:

1. The treatment itself has no relevant biological activity

One early consideration in the Gard case was whether NRT would cross the blood-brain barrier. If it didn't, it would be futile. However, by July, it was accepted that the medicine would be able to reach the brain. That argument failed.

The dominant ground for a judgment of futility in the High Court Decision was that there was no direct evidence that such therapy would have any effect on Charlie's condition (the *RRM2B*-related form of mitochondrial DNA depletion syndrome (MDDS)) because it had never been tried in humans or animal models.

The only evidence Hirano produced was from patients with another related disorder (the *TK2*-related form of MDDS). These studies were small (18 patients) with modest results, and no blinded controlled trials had been conducted. There was, however, a physiological rationale for believing that, as Hirano claimed, the chances of improvement in Charlie's condition were 'low, but not zero.' Hirano said that 'were Charlie in the US, he would treat him.'

Remarkably, Judge Francis immediately concluded: 'The long and the short of Dr I's [Hirano's] evidence is that there is no scientific evidence of any prospect of any improvement in a human with RRM2B strain of MDDS. While there were some reasons to be hopeful that it might make a modest difference to life expectancy, it almost certainly could not undo structural brain damage.' (Para 21)[2]

If a treatment might increase life expectancy, then it is a value judgment, not a medical or scientific judgment, whether such treatment is worthwhile. In my view (and that of Peter Singer), Hirano did present evidence that the treatment might make a modest difference to life expectancy (although the evidence was not strong), and Judge Francis appears to have accepted this evidence. To accept it, and to say that 'there is no scientific evidence of any prospect of any improvement' is either self-contradictory or conceals a value judgment to the effect that, for a patient in Charlie's condition, a longer life is not an improvement. If such a concealed value judgment lay behind Judge Francis's decision, it should have been made explicit and defended.

More importantly, as I will shortly argue, there was no evidence presented of structural brain damage.

In early July, President Trump and the Pope became involved, and Hirano and six other world experts wrote with new evidence of activity in 'cultured human cells with *RRM2B* mutations.' They also urged reconsideration of the scientific plausibility of treatment. The evidence they presented supported Hirano's claim that the chances of it working were nonzero and thus, from a biological perspective, it was not definitely futile.

2. Irreversible damage

Indeed, following the expert report, the argument shifted to a second and distinct ground on which treatment for Charlie might be futile. Although an agent might have biological utility,

---

[a]I developed these arguments first in a blog with Peter Singer.[3]

features about a particular patient might mean that it will not work on that patient. It was the alleged fact that Charlie had suffered irreversible brain damage around January that led the Court in April to find treatment was futile.

After muscle scans were performed in July, there was subsequent general agreement that Charlie's condition was irreversible. When Charlie Gard was born in August 2016, he had normal muscle and brain function. The injury came on gradually as cells became starved of energy. It is not clear at what precise point his damage became irreversible and the window of opportunity for a trial of treatment closed. In December, he began fitting. This is a sign of brain injury, but not necessarily brain cell death. In January, his fitting increased. At that time, a scan showed that, although Charlie's brain function was abnormal, its structure appeared normal.[2,4] Justice Francis, in his final judgment, referred to 'structural brain damage'. This was an error. As the Court of Appeal itself noted, 'at paragraph 79 he [Justice Francis himself] stated that an MRI scan "appeared to show no structural damage".' (Para 42)[4] Nevertheless, the Court of Appeal ruled this error was irrelevant because 'Charlie had sustained a loss of neurones' based on 'the pattern of regular seizures'. (Para 42)[4]

No doubt Charlie had sustained 'a loss of neurones', but the crux of the matter was how many neurones had been lost, and whether all or some of this brain damage was reversible. No argument or evidence was presented that 'regular seizures' constitute irrefutable evidence of irreversible brain damage. Hirano did not accept this, nor did the Italian specialist who attended in July. No actual EEG evidence was presented in the High Court of irreversibility, such as flat line. Indeed, seizures indicate the brain is still functioning, albeit in a very disordered way. No definitive tests such as a brain biopsy appear to have been performed.

So, while Hirano, the Italian expert and Charlie's parents eventually (in July) reached a consensus that Charlie's condition was irreversible, this was not a consensus that Charlie had irreversible brain damage. It was a muscle scan (ordered by the Italian expert) that was the deciding factor.

Even as late as July, Hirano and the Italian expert did not appear to accept that the MRI scan of Charlie's brain showed total irreversible damage. On that ground alone, they appeared to believe a trial would be reasonable.[5] This implies that grounds of irreversible brain damage would not have applied 6 months earlier, in January, based on their reasoning.

We cannot know exactly when Charlie's injury became irreversible. During the period when there was uncertainty, it would have been reasonable to employ a limited 3-month trial of experimental therapy or to employ a more definitive test.

PROBABILITY TOO LOW

If we reject the argument that further treatment was not in Charlie's interests because it would have been futile, it would still be possible to argue that treatment was not in Charlie's interests because the chance of improvement, although nonzero, was too low to justify the suffering it would inflict.

In these circumstances, what chance of improvement is too low? 1%? 0.1%? I have already given five arguments for why a trial might be construed as being in Charlie's interests and the chances not too low.

Partly, the answer depends also on the likelihood of the treatment causing suffering to the patient, and the severity and duration of that suffering. Statements by Great Ormond Street Hospital, which I outline in the next section, cast doubt on whether Charlie could experience anything at all, including pain.[6] If that were correct, he would not have suffered if subjected to a trial. If there had been a reasonable likelihood that he was capable of experiencing pain, careful analgesia and sedation would have been able to limit the extent of his suffering.[7]

Once we are clear about the probability and nature of the suffering Charlie would have experienced, if treated, the remainder of the argument is ethical. It requires us to ask: what risk of suffering is worth taking, given that without treatment Charlie would certainly die, and with treatment there was a small chance that he would live? If the probability that the treatment would cause severe suffering or prolonged suffering were very low, and the treatment were not paid for from public funds, even an extremely low chance that the treatment would succeed would have sufficed to make it reasonable to treat Charlie.

BEST OUTCOME IS A LIFE NOT WORTH LIVING

Justice Francis describes the basis for his decision:

'The relevant legal principles which guide the exercise of my discretion are well settled.... The judge must decide what is in the child's best interests. In making that decision, the welfare of the child is paramount, and the judge must look at the question from the assumed point of view of the child ... The term "best interests" encompasses medical, emotional, and all other welfare issues.' (para 12-13)[2]

We can call this a 'welfarist view' of the worth of life because it is related to a judgment over expected welfare or wellbeing. While this account is defensible, it is inadequate, as it does not specify what constitutes wellbeing or where the line is to be drawn. This is a feature of existing legal discussions of the worth of life, as we shall see. Justice Francis claims that this test is 'objective' and not subjective. But it is unsatisfactory that a baby lives or dies on the basis of a test which cannot be defined and rests ultimately with the intuitions and feelings of the sitting judge.

The welfarist view entails that, even if the treatment were 'successful', the best outcome that could be achieved is still not one worth aiming for either in terms of length or quality of life.

The parents' own medical expert, Dr L, said:

'The nature of Charlie's condition means that he is likely to continue to deteriorate, that he is likely to remain immobile, that he will exhibit severe cognitive impairment, that he will remain dependent on ventilatory support to maintain respiration, will continue to need to be tube fed and that he will always be dependent on mechanical ventilation to maintain life.' (para 91)[2]

Judge Francis concluded after this piece of evidence:

'... Dr L's conclusions coincided with the reports to which I have already referred in this judgment.... 'Accordingly, the entire highly experienced UK team, all those who provided second opinions and the consultant instructed by the parents in these proceedings share a common view that further treatment would be futile.' (para 93)[2]

Judge Francis appears to overlook the fact that Dr L was offering a view of the natural history of the disease, without improvement; but putting that aside, Dr L's evidence tends to show, not that treatment would be futile in a medical sense, but that if it were successful, Charlie would lead a life of such poor quality that it would not be worth living. That raises an ethical question: is a life with cognitive impairment, immobility, tube feeding and ventilatory support one that is not worth living, from the individual's own perspective?

There are three issues with this welfarist account of the worth of life based on dependency and disability which need to be addressed before it can be deployed.

Firstly, it seems to suggest that, at some point, disability makes life not worth living, and that the severely disabled would be better off dead, from their own perspective. Disability groups may well disagree. Some people who are quadriplegic on a ventilator with spinal muscular atrophy find their lives worth living. Many severely disabled people find their own lives worth living.[8,9]

It runs the risk of being accused of being 'ableist', discriminating against those with disability. Perhaps, for this reason, where the line lies on this account has been left fuzzy.

One way in which humans differ from nonhuman animals is in certain abilities. But nobody cites the lack of abilities in nonhuman animals as a reason to think that their lives are not worth living from their own perspective – abilities are an irrelevant consideration. Nor do we consider the fact that some humans have significantly greater abilities than average to mean their lives are more worth living than those who are only average – again, abilities are an irrelevant consideration. Why then should the lack of certain abilities be an important factor for a human over whether they have or do not have a life which is worth living?

Secondly, disability is instrumentally bad: it is not in itself what matters. Rather, as Judge Francis acknowledged, it is wellbeing or welfare that is intrinsically good. As I have argued elsewhere,[10,11] whether deafness or paralysis reduces wellbeing is context-dependent. How bad functional disabilities are will depend on the social context and state of technology.

Indeed, Justice Hedley, in another case (that of Charlotte Wyatt, which was cited as the basis of the Gard decision), said that 'Best interests must be given a generous interpretation'[3] but, although he referred to the broader concept of best interests as including nonmedical interests, he did not go further, saying simply that 'The infinite variety of the human condition never ceases to surprise and it is that fact that defeats any attempt to be more precise in a definition of best interests'.[12]

Thirdly, the bar of a life worth living has been set very low – even at minimal consciousness, as the case of M illustrates. M contracted viral encephalitis back in 2003, leaving her in a minimally conscious state. Her family petitioned a court to remove her artificial nutrition and hydration on the basis of her previously expressed wishes. However, the judge, using the 'balance sheet' approach used in the Gard case and other cases, came up with the following view:

> 'M does experience pain and discomfort, and her disability severely restricts what she can do. Having considered all the evidence, however, I find that she does have some positive experiences and importantly that there is a reasonable prospect that those experiences can be extended by a planned programme of increased stimulation'.[13]

M had profound cognitive impairment. She was nearly unconscious. Despite her family's evidence that she would not want to live in such a state, the judge decided that it was in her best interests to live with such profound disability.

Pleasure and pain are important. According to this view, it is pleasure and pain which are highly important factors in deciding whether life is worth living.

So evidently, the bar that Charlie Gard would have to jump to reach a life worth living was not very high, at least in the view of some judges, and it was mainly determined in that case by the balance of pain and pleasure.

We need to tether the line of a life more closely to wellbeing, and specify more what constitutes wellbeing, rather than the vague, open-ended accounts employed so far in law. Philosophers Derek Parfit and James Griffin describe three theories of wellbeing: the Hedonistic, Desire Fulfilment and Objective List theories.[14,15] According to Hedonistic theories, what makes life go well is pleasure and happiness, and what makes life go badly is pain and unhappiness. According to Desire Fufilment theories, what makes life go well is being able to satisfy desires, and what makes it go badly are frustrated desires.

Parfit explains Objective List theories in the following way:

> '[C]ertain things are good or bad for people, whether or not these people want to have the good things or avoid the bad things. The good things might include moral goodness, rational activity, the development of one's abilities, having children and being a good parent, knowledge and the

awareness of true beauty. The bad things might include being betrayed, manipulated, slandered, deceived, being deprived of liberty and dignity, and enjoying either sadistic pleasure, or aesthetic pleasure in what is in fact ugly.[14]

Objective List theories can be extended.[16] Other items might include love, deep and varied personal relationships, originality, creativity, autonomy, engagement with nature and sex.

Each of the three accounts of wellbeing – Hedonistic, Desire Fulfilment and Objective List theories – has some plausibility. Parfit concludes that an adequate account of wellbeing must accord weight to all valuable mental states, desire satisfaction and objectively valuable activity.[17] It may be best not only to engage in activities that possess objective value, but to also want to engage in such activities and to derive pleasure from them.

Given the wide disagreement about what constitutes a good life and a life worth living, the least controversial account of a life not worth living is one which is not worth living on all three accounts:

1. balance of pain over a pleasure;
2. greater desire frustration than fulfilment;
3. lack of any objective goods or objectively valuable activity in life.

Disability will be relevant to these three criteria but we cannot say what its precise effect will be on wellbeing outside of the specific context, and especially outside the specific social and technological context. A life with loving and devoted parents may tip the balance of pleasure over pain.

The pervading presence of pain in such an account is important. It is on the basis of unrelenting pain that some people believe life with severe dystrophic epidermolysis bullosa (where the skin peels off and death occurs very early in life) and Lesch-Nyhan disease (characterised by intellectual disability and painful self-mutilation) are sometimes said to be lives which are not worth living.

There was considerable disagreement about the extent to which Charlie Gard was actually suffering. In the High Court Decision in April,

> *'Professor A said that Charlie is likely to have the conscious experience of pain. Professor A expressed the important need to weigh up the potential benefit of the smallest of chances (her views being that there were no chances) against the continued pain of intensive care, ventilator support and so forth. She said that it was her view and the view of other members of the team that Charlie is suffering and that that outweighs the tiny theoretical chance there may be of effective treatment. She said that she did not regard his pain of being of a low level of suffering, but something more significant.'* (Para 114)[2]

Yet a statement released by GOSH in July stated that

> *'so far as can be discerned after many months of encephalopathy, [he lives] without any awareness. At the moment, he is on a low dose of oral morphine. Before that was started quite recently, all of those caring for him at GOSH hoped very much that Charlie did not experience pain. They did so in the knowledge that if he did not, it was because he had no experience at all because he was beyond experience.'*[6]

So even though Charlie was thought to be experiencing pain in April, low dose morphine was only started much later. Clearly there was uncertainty about how much pain he was experiencing. Indeed, it was uncertain whether he was suffering pain at all.

Pain is extremely difficult to determine in the absence of report. There are some conditions, like brain death and permanent unconsciousness, in which there is a reasonable consensus that life is not worth living. But for conditions like minimally conscious state or other severe cognitive impairment, there can be reasonable disagreement. I don't know if it is worth living in a minimally conscious state. I have never read or heard reliable reports from people who have lived in that state. I have written that it might be kind of living hell,[18,19] but it might not be. We don't know.

It will always be difficult to make life and death decisions on the value of experiences which are necessarily subjective.

When there is reasonable disagreement about whether some state is worth living in, or a chance is worth taking, we should defer to other factors, like the person's own past wishes or values, or those of the parents whose child it is. Just as we should have deferred to the wishes of M, as the court did in the similar case of Briggs,[20] we should defer to the wishes of parents if we are unsure whether the life of their child has crossed the line of not being worth living, not because they must be right, but just because there is reasonable disagreement.

I personally have a high threshold for a life that is worth living, so I am inclined to agree with the judgment that the kind of life Dr L described is not worth living. Many people, however, do not share my view. They would hold that, as long as Charlie was conscious and capable of experiencing pleasure, then his life was worth living. Indeed, this seems to be ground used by one judge in the W versus M case to order that a woman who was minimally conscious should not be allowed to die, despite her past wishes.[13]

Although I disagree with the view we have just described, and with the view of the previously mentioned judge in W versus M, I accept that the claim that such a life is a fate worse than death is not self-evident, and so stands in need of justification. In the Charlie Gard case, no justification was attempted.

Conclusion

The doctors and courts accepted the view that the proposed experimental treatment was not in Charlie Gard's interests. This argument has a number of different versions, but all are, in this case, problematic. Moreover, there are a number of arguments that it was in his best interests to receive a trial of NRT.

Charlie Gard's parents requested permission to take Charlie to the US because they saw this as giving Charlie a chance at life. If permission had been granted, they would have taken him to a world-class centre where he could be treated by a world-leading expert who believed there was a nonzero chance of some improvement. They had raised the funds to pay for his travel and treatment, and so there was no argument from distributive justice against their doing so. On the basis of the evidence and argument presented, I conclude that their request was reasonable.

At the end of the Today programme on BBC, when I was interviewed in July near the end of Charlie's life, the presenter concluded by asking me, in a forceful kind of way: "So you think all these doctors and all these Courts are wrong?" I replied, "Yes."

Everything I have seen and learnt since then confirms that judgment.

Of course, I could still be wrong. We don't have all the relevant facts. At many points in the case of Charlie Gard, I wondered whether I was right to pursue my line of argument, especially when someone I know and respect so much as Dominic Wilkinson, who is practising medicine at the coal face, thought so differently. We continued to debate and both of us found where we disagreed; we were both prepared to revise our views if certain facts came to light. For me, this has been the most important lived experience of practical ethics in my life. To be engaging in dialogue and argument with an equal whom you respect and to find your own and their thinking advancing is perhaps the main aim of practical ethics.

As we have together written, disagreement in medicine is inevitable.[21] Conflict should not be. We have to find a way to live with empirical uncertainty and value pluralism. It is ethics, not science, that will enable us.

A happy ending postscript

In practical ethics, it is important to evaluate all the possible alternatives, not a selected range. Moreover, most real life ethical dilemmas don't have happy endings like Hollywood scripts. There are usually a series of tradeoffs that we wish we didn't have to make. The best option is rarely, if ever, the perfect option.

But the case of Charlie Gard, and the hypothetical case of SMA discussed in Chapter 9, are cases where there could have been a happy ending, one in which everyone is a winner. Both SMA and *RR2MB*-related MDDS are genetic disorders caused by mutations in each of the parent's genes. When you have one copy of the gene, it doesn't have any effect (it is recessive). But when a child is conceived with one copy from each parent, that child has the devastating genetic disorder. All of us carry three to four recessive genetic mutations such that, if we meet a partner with the same one, we have a one in four chance of having a child with a severe genetic condition (like SMA, *RR2MB*-related MDDS, cystic fibrosis, thalassaemia or one of more than 300 other conditions).

Thankfully, science progresses at an exponential rate, and there are therapies like nusinersin which can have some impact on disorders like SMA. In the future, gene editing of the early embryo could be used to correct the abnormality at the very earliest stage of life. It would be a genetic cure for babies like Charlie. But it would require in-vitro fertilisation and genetic testing of the embryo. In the future, it will be possible to test the whole genome of the embryo and scan for diseases like this. However, at present, gene editing is too risky to attempt on human beings and is banned in many parts of the world for treatment purposes, including the UK.

Nonetheless, there is already a fairytale solution available right now. Parents like Chris Gard and Connie Yates, or our hypothetical SMA parents Stefan and Janeczka, need never have a child afflicted by a severe genetic disorder. What could be done right now is whole genome carrier testing. Couples thinking of having a child could have their genome tested for the 300 or so recessive mutations. If they found they both carried a similar one, they could go on to artificial reproduction (IVF), form a number of embryos and select a healthy embryo without a major genetic condition. This is routinely done for common genetic disorders like cystic fibrosis and thalassaemia, where people know they are at risk. The Gards could have this for their next pregnancy. However, it is not routinely available.

Carrier testing could be introduced. We choose not to. That is an ethical decision. It could allow healthy children to be born instead of children who will, at best, have lives dominated by suffering and severe disability.

The only good argument against it is resources: that it is not cost-effective. Distributive justice precludes its widespread introduction. I doubt those arguments can succeed. But that is a topic for another book.

Without a doubt, if people wish to pay for their own carrier testing, doctors ought to support that wish. There is no good ethical argument against it. And they ought to be made aware of this life-changing option.

References

1. Savulescu, J. (2017) Is it in Charlie Gard's best interest to die? *Lancet*, 389, 1868-1869.
2. *Great Ormond Street Hospital v Yates & Ors [2017] EWHC 972 (Fam) (11 April 2017)*.
3. Savulescu, J. & Singer, P. (2017). 'Unpicking what we mean by best interests in light of Charlie Gard.' From <http://blogs.bmj.com/bmj/2017/08/02/unpicking-what-we-mean-by-best-interests-in-light-of-charlie-gard/>.
4. Yates and Gard v GOSH and Charles Gard [2017] EWCA Civ 410, 20.
5. Edwards J. *Charlie Gard: Parents end legal fight after latest MRI scan*. Legal Loop. http://www.legalloop.co.uk/charlie-gard-parents-end-legal-fight-latest-mri-scan/. Accessed 28 July 2017.
6. Gollop K. GOSH'S Position Statement Hearing on 13 July 2017. http://www.gosh.nhs.uk/file/23611/download?token=aTPZchww. Accessed 28 July 2017.

7. Truog RD. The United Kingdom Sets Limits on Experimental Treatments: The Case of Charlie Gard. *JAMA* 2017 doi:10.1001/jama.2017.10410.

8. http://notdeadyetuk.org/about/.

9. http://www.worldhealthinnovationsummit.com/blog/2016/07/26/health-why-severely-disabled-lives-matter-too/.

10. Savulescu, J. & Kahane, G. (2011) Disability: a welfarist approach. *Clinical Ethics* 6:45-51.

11. Kahane, G. & Savulescu, J. (2009) The Welfarist Account of Disability. In *Disability and Disadvantage* eds A. Cureton and K. Brownlee. Oxford: Oxford University Press, pp. 14–53.

12. *Portsmouth NHS Trust v Wyatt [2005] 1 F.L.R. 21.*

13. *W v. M [2011] EWHC 2443 [Fam].*

14. Parfit, D. *Reasons and persons.* Oxford University Press, 1984.

15. Griffin, J. (1986). *Well-being: its meaning, measurement, and moral importance.* Clarendon Press.

16. Nussbaum M. (2011). *Creating capabilities: the human development approach.* Harvard University Press, pp 33-34.

17. Parfit D. *Reasons and Persons.* Oxford: Oxford University Press, 1984:502.

18. Savulescu, J & Kahane, G. (2009). Brain-damage and the moral significance of consciousness'. *J Med Philo* 34:6-26.

19. Wilkinson, D & Savulescu, J. (2013). Commentary: is it better to be minimally conscious than vegetative? *J Med Ethics* 39:557–558.

20. *Briggs v Briggs [2016] EWCOP 53.*

21. Wilkinson, D., Barclay, S., Savulescu, J. 2018. Disagreement, mediation, arbitration: resolving disputes about medical treatment. *The Lancet* 391 (10137):2302-5.

Page numbers followed by "*f*" indicate figures, "*t*" indicate tables, and "*b*" indicate boxes.

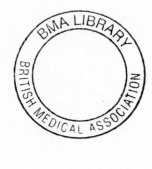